Copyright © 2021 -All rights reserved.

No part of this book may be reproduced or transmitted in any form or by any means, electronic or mechanical, including photocopying and recording, or by any information storage and retrieval system, without permission in writing from the publisher. This is a work of fiction. Names, places, characters and incidents are either the product of the author's imagination or are used fictitiously, and any resemblance to any actual persons, living or dead, organizations, events or locales is entirely coincidental. The unauthorized reproduction or distribution of this copyrighted work is ilegal.

Please note the information contained within this document is for educational and entertainment purposes only. All effort has been executed to present accurate, up to date, reliable, complete information. No warranties of any kind are declared or implied. Readers acknowledge that the author is not engaged in the rendering of legal, financial, medical, or professional advice. The content within this book has been derived from various sources. Please consult a licensed professional before attempting any techniques outlined in this book. By reading this document, the reader agrees that under no circumstances is the author responsible for any losses, direct or indirect, that are incurred as a result of the use of the information contained within this document, including, but not limited to, errors, omissions, or inaccuracies.

CONTENTS

- **INTRODUCTION** 7
- **CHAPTER 1: BREAKFAST** 10
  - Vanilla Pancakes 10
  - Veggie Turkey Smash 10
  - Paprika Shrimp 10
  - Breakfast Pizza 11
  - Breakfast Sweet Pepper Hash 11
  - Pork Breakfast Sausages 11
  - Potato Breakfast Mix 12
  - Breakfast Veggie Casserole 12
  - Cheddar Jalapeno Breakfast Sausages 13
  - Breakfast Veggie Salad 13
  - Breakfast Pork and Avocado Mix 13
  - Eggplant Pate with Breadcrumbs 14
  - Red Beans with the Sweet Peas 14
  - Nutritious Burrito Bowl 15
  - Quinoa Curry 15
  - Ham Pitta Pockets 16
  - Breakfast Meatloaf 16
  - Breakfast Sweet Pepper Rounds 16
  - Breakfast Cauliflower Hash 17
  - Healthy Low Carb Walnut Zucchini Bread 17
  - Bacon & Cheese Frittata 18
  - Low-Carb Hash Brown Breakfast Casserole 18
  - Asparagus Smoked Salmon 19
  - Onion Broccoli Quiche 19
  - Thyme Sausage Squash 20
  - Tasty Greek Style Breakfast 20
- **CHAPTER 2: LUNCH** 21
  - Lime Chicken with Savoy Cabbage 21
  - Middle Eastern Lamb Zucchini Casserole 21
  - Ginger Steak Broccoli 21
  - BLT Chicken Salad 22
  - Figs and Goat Cheese-Stuffed Chicken 22
  - Carne Asada 23
  - Amazing Pulled Pork 23
  - Braised Pork Belly 24
  - Peppercorn Short Ribs 24
  - Spicy Italian Sausage and Zucchini Noodles 24
  - Meaty Cauliflower Lasagna 25
  - Chili Verde 25
  - Tandoori Salmon with Fresh Cucumber Salad 26
- **CHAPTER 3: DINNER** 27
  - Hungarian Mushroom Soup 27
  - Curried Cauliflower 27
  - Cheese Stuffed and Pesto Eggplants 27
  - Creamy Vegan Broccoli Soup 28
  - The Ultimate Bacon Meatloaf 28
  - Cheese and Mushroom Stuffed Chicken Rolls 28
  - Tasty Short Ribs 29
  - Garlic Butter Turkey Breasts 29
  - Creamy Salmon and Dill 30

Shrimps Alfredo	30
Mediterranean Fresh Tuna	30
Low Carb Seafood and Sausage Gumbo	31

CHAPTER 4: SIDE DISHES 32

Zucchini Pasta	32
Chinese Broccoli	32
Slow Cooker Spaghetti Squash	32
Mushroom Stew	33
Cabbage Steaks	33
Mashed Cauliflower	33
Bacon-Wrapped Cauliflower	34
Cauliflower Casserole	34
Cauliflower Rice	35
Curry Cauliflower	35
Garlic Cauliflower Steaks	35
Zucchini Gratin	36
Eggplant Gratin	36
Moroccan Eggplant Mash	36
Sautéed Bell Peppers	37

CHAPTER 5: SNACKS AND APPETIZERS 38

Chicken Bites	38
Paprika Almonds	38
Mixed Nuts	38
Beef and Zucchini Wraps	38
Cauliflower Bites	39
Cheese Sticks	39
Eggplant Bread	39
Almond Granola	40
Chili Walnuts	40
Pork Bites	40
Turkey Meatballs	41
Tomato Salmon Meatballs	41
Pecans Bowl	41
Sausage Dip	42
Butter Pork Ribs	42

CHAPTER 6: FISH AND SEAFOOD 43

Mahi Mahi Taco Wraps	43
Shrimp Scampi	43
Shrimp Tacos	44
Fish Curry	44
Salmon with Creamy Lemon Sauce	44
Salmon with Lemon-Caper Sauce	45
Spicy Barbecue Shrimp	45
Lemon Dill Halibut	46
Coconut Cilantro Curry Shrimp	46
Shrimp in Marinara Sauce	47
Garlic Shrimp	47
Poached Salmon	48
Lemon Pepper Tilapia	48
Clam Chowder	48
Soy-Ginger Steamed Pompano	49

CHAPTER 7: POULTRY 50

Chicken Noodle Soup	50
Chicken Enchilada Casserole	50

Chicken Basque 51
Chicken Curry 51
Chicken & Pumpkin Chili 52
Maple Chicken & Veggies 52
Chicken Parmesan Soup 53
Sweet Spicy Chicken 53
Chicken Cordon Bleu Soup 53
Honey Garlic Chicken 54
Chicken & Corn Chowder 54
Moroccan Chicken 55
Quinoa Chicken Primavera 56
Chicken with Mint Garlic Sauce & Lentils 56
Orange Chicken 57
Aromatic Jalapeno Wings 57
Barbeque Chicken Wings 58
Saucy Duck 58
Chicken Roux Gumbo 59
Cider-Braised Chicken 59
Chunky Chicken Salsa 59
Dijon Chicken 60
Chicken Thighs with Vegetables 60
Chicken Dipped in Tomatillo Sauce 61
Chicken with Lemon Parsley Butter 61
Paprika Chicken 61
Rotisserie Chicken 62
Chicken Ginger Curry 62
Thai Chicken Curry 63

CHAPTER 8: MEAT 64
Mexican Lamb Fillet 64
Beef Mac & Cheese 64
Beef and Scallions Bowl 64
Balsamic Beef 65
Simple Pork Chop Casserole 65
Balsamic Lamb Chops 65
Lamb and Cabbage 66
Lavender and Orange Lamb 66
Beer Sausages 66
Hamburger Style Stuffing 67
Classic Pork Adobo 67
Pork Ragu With Basil 68
Indian Style Cardamom Pork 68
Beef with Spinach 68
Beef with Peas and Corn 69
Barbacoa Lamb 69
Lamb with Mint & Green Beans 69
Succulent Lamb 70
Tarragon Lamb & Beans 70
BBQ Beef Burritos 71
Cheeseburger & Bacon Pie 71
Italian Meatballs & Zoodles 72
Italian Meatloaf 72
Beef Bourguignon with Carrot Noodles 73
Beef & Broccoli 73
Beef Ribs 74

- Braised Oxtails ... 74
- Brisket & Onions ... 75
- Italian Ragu ... 75
- Mississippi Pot Roast ... 75

CHAPTER 9: VEGETABLE MEALS ... 77
- Aloo Gobi ... 77
- Jackfruit Carnitas ... 77
- Baked Beans ... 77
- Brussels Sprouts Curry ... 78
- Jambalaya ... 78
- Mushroom-Kale Stroganoff ... 79
- Sloppy Joe Filling ... 79
- Hoppin' John ... 80
- African Sweet Potato Stew ... 80
- Sweet-and-Sour Tempeh ... 80
- Delightful Dal ... 81
- Moroccan Chickpea Stew ... 81
- Tex-Mex Taco Filling ... 82
- Ratatouille ... 82
- Cauliflower Bolognese ... 83
- Vegan Cauliflower Rice and Beans ... 83
- Tomatoes Aubergines ... 84
- Bacon Brussels Sprouts ... 84
- Egg and Broccoli Casserole ... 85
- Delicious Garden Frittata ... 85
- Broccoli Cheese Casserole ... 86
- Chicken Butter Mushrooms ... 86
- Brunch Florentine ... 86
- Fire Roasted Tomato Soup ... 87
- Vegetable Cheese Frittata ... 87
- Beefy Vegetable Soup ... 88
- Zucchini Lasagna ... 88
- Pumpkin and Coconut Soup ... 89
- Crustless Spinach Quiche ... 89
- Vegetarian Tikka Masala ... 89

CHAPTER 10: SOUPS ... 91
- Creamy Chicken Soup ... 91
- Mexican Chicken Soup ... 91
- Thai-Inspired Chicken Soup ... 91
- Spicy Pepper Chicken Soup ... 92
- Turkey + Herbs Soup ... 92
- Beefy Chili ... 93
- Shredded Pork Chili ... 93
- Beef Minestrone ... 94
- Cream of Broccoli-Cauliflower Soup ... 94
- Cheesy Cauliflower Chowder w/ Bacon ... 95
- Ham + Pumpkin Soup ... 95
- Cream of Zucchini Soup ... 96
- Tomato Soup ... 96
- Vegetable Korma (Stew) ... 96

CHAPTER 11: DESSERTS ... 98
- Raspberry Yogurt ... 98
- Banana Bread ... 98
- Rice Pudding with Mixed Berries ... 98

Banana Raisin Bread Pudding ... 99
Chocolate Peanut Butter Cups ... 99
Flourless Chocolate Brownies ... 99
Crème Brulee ... 100
Chocolate Cheese Cake ... 100
Peanut Butter Pudding ... 100
Coconut Yogurt ... 100
Delicious Pumpkin Custard ... 101
Lemon Blueberry Cake ... 101
Tasty Lemon Cake ... 102
Chocolate Cake ... 102
Coconut Raspberry Cake ... 103
APPENDIX : RECIPES INDEX ... 104

INTRODUCTION

A keto diet isn't one that you can keep going on and off. It will take your body some time to get adjusted and for ketosis to set in. This process could take anywhere between two to seven days. It depends on the level of activity, body type, and food you are eating. If you start exercising on an
empty stomach, this will help in inducing ketosis rather quickly. Start restricting your carb consumption to less than 20g per day and be mindful of the amount of water that you are consuming.

All the recipes that you need have been provided in this book! You needn't worry about having to search for recipes. The recipes provided in this book have been divided into different categories for the convenience of the reader. So, you have got recipes for other courses. Once you get the hang of all the things you can and cannot eat, you can start experimenting on your own. All that you will need to do will be to plan your meals.

There are various mobile applications that you can make use for tracking your carbohydrate intake. There are paid and free applications as well. These apps will help you in keeping track of your total carbohydrate and fiber intake. However, you won't be able to track your net carb intake. MyFitnessPal is one of the popular apps. You just need to open the app store on your smartphone, and you can select an app from the various available apps.

Calories do matter. There are different reasons that you will need to be mindful of while counting calories. You will need to eat correctly and ensure that your body doesn't have a severe calories deficit. Also, don't indulge in snacks that aren't good for you. While on a keto diet, you usually have to worry about the calories you are consuming due to all the fats and proteins that you will be consuming for filling yourself up. If you exercise regularly, make sure that you consume sufficient calories and that your body isn't experiencing a massive calorie deficit.

To state it simply, you can eat fat. Your body will need to be in a state of caloric deficit for losing weight. This means that calories are an essential marker at the end of the day. If you start consuming too much fat, then this will turn the caloric deficit into a surplus. It isn't easy to overeat while on a high-fat diet like keto, but it is still possible. Make use of apps for keeping track of your macros and check the amount of fats, proteins, and carbs you should be consuming. The quantity of weight that you will drop will depend on you. If you add exercise to your daily routine, then the weight loss will be greater. If you cut down on foods that stall weight loss, then this will speed up the process. For instance, completely cutting out things like artificial sweeteners, dairy and wheat products, and other related products will help speed up your weight loss. During the first two weeks of the keto diet, you will lose all the excess water weight. Ketosis has a diuretic result on the body, and you might end up losing a couple of pounds within the first few days of this diet. After this, your body will adapt itself to burning fats for generating energy instead of carbs.

The most common way you can tell whether your body is in ketosis or not is by using Ketostix. These can be found in any local pharmacy. However, it would be best if you kept in mind that they can be entirely inaccurate. Usually, they will give you an idea of whether ketosis has been induced or not. If the stick turns purple or pink, this shows that your body is producing ketones. If it is a darker color, this could mean that you are dehydrated and that ketone levels in your urine are quite concentrated. Ketostix will help in measuring the levels of acetone present in your urine. Ketones, when unused, produce acetone. The Ketostix helps measure the acetone present in your urine, and these are the unused ketones present. The ketones used by your brain and body for generating energy are known as Beta-Hydroxybutyrate (BHB), and

the Ketostix doesn't measure these. If you want an accurate measure of the ketone levels in your body, you should use a blood ketone meter. These will show you the actual number of ketones present in the bloodstream and aren't easily influenced by hydration or it lack.

To put it simply, Ketosis is the state that the body would be induced into when you don't consume any carbohydrates. The body will start making use of fats to provide energy. So, fats, including body fats, would be the primary source of fuel. It not only healthier, but it is also a more efficient source of fuel for the brain. You might be wondering how energy is generated from all the fats present. In the state of Ketosis, the liver helps break down the fat molecules and produces ketones. These ketones are made use of for providing the necessary energy. How does all this help in losing weight? When there is a deficit of calories, the body starts making use of the stored reserves of fat for providing the energy it needs. The human body has been designed so that they have reserves of fat in case our food intake decreases. These fat reserves are hardly ever made use of and lead to weight gain. Reducing the calorie intake by cutting down on carbs helps in losing their extra kilos.

Macro is the term that is usually used for macronutrients. The three main macronutrients are fats, proteins, and carbs. As mentioned earlier, calories don't matter. Though, it would be better if you keep track of these at the beginning. It will enable you to see how you are doing on a diet. You will genuinely be surprised about the amount of carbs that we end up consuming unknowingly. If you have come to a standstill in your weight loss, then tracking macros will be helpful. You will be able to pinpoint the different things in your diet that might be causing this. You will start thinking in terms of grams when you start tracking your macros. You shouldn't think in terms of % but think in terms of grams. For instance, a lot of people think that 75% fat, 20% protein, and 5% carbs are good. However, that's not the case. Grams will help you in getting an accurate description of what you are eating. You needn't worry if you are off by a bit on your macros; it isn't a big deal. There is a wiggle room for about 10-15 grams of fats as well as proteins in most cases. You needn't worry if you go a little over or a little under on some days. If you keep track of your calories and it isn't too much in deficit, you are doing fine.

During the initial phase of the keto diet, you might experience mild headaches and feel a little low on energy as well. Ketosis has a diuretic effect on the individual, and this increases the urge to urinate more than usual. Added to this, your body is burning up the glycogen stores, and you have got a minor problem on your hands. The electrolytes are being pushed out of your body. So, you will need to replace them. Keep yourself fully hydrated. Add a little salt to your food. Consume plenty of broths and have lots of water. The transition into ketosis will be quite simple, and you can make it easy on yourself by staying hydrated.

Your bowel movements might change while starting on keto. You might or might not experience constipation. At this time are a few things that you can do for restoring normalcy to your bowel movements. Add in a magnesium supplement, drink lots of water, a tbsp. of coconut oil will help, if you eat nuts, then stop doing so for a while, consume fibrous vegetables, chia, or flax seeds, and try some coffee or some tea.

You can consume alcohol while on the ketogenic diet. However, be mindful of the amount of alcohol you consume. Alcohol is an excellent source of carbs to creep into your diet. You should concentrate on the liquor you are drinking. Wine, beer, and different cocktails have carbs in them. So, clear liquor would be a safe bet. However, stay away from all sorts of flavored liquors since they have got carbs in them as well.

You might have reached a standstill in your weight loss. There are a lot of reasons that could contribute to this. You can do a couple of things for resuming your weight loss. Cut down a few things from your diet, or you could change your eating pattern as well. Here are a few suggestions that you can make use of. You can try any of the following strategies. You can cut down on dairy, increase your fat intake, and decrease the intake of carbs. You may also stop consuming nuts, cut out gluten, no artificial sweeteners, watch out for additional carbs, cut down on processed foods, and switch to measuring yourself instead of weighing yourself.

CHAPTER 1: BREAKFAST

Vanilla Pancakes

Preparation Time: 15 Minutes Cooking Time: 2 Hours Servings: 6
Ingredients:
- 1 cup coconut flour
- Two eggs, beaten
- One teaspoon baking powder
- One tablespoon vanilla extract

Directions:
- One tablespoon ghee
- ½ cup almond milk
- ¾ teaspoon salt
- ¼ teaspoon nutmeg

1. Whisk the eggs with the coconut flour and baking powder in the mixing bowl.
2. Add vanilla extract and ghee. Then add milk, salt, and nutmeg.
3. Stir the pancake mixture carefully until smooth.
4. Pour the pancake batter into the slow cooker and close the lid. Cook the pancake for 2 hours on High.
5. When the pancake is cooked, cut it into servings and serve. Enjoy!

Nutrition: Calories 173, Fat 10.4, Fiber 8.5, Carbs 15.3, Protein 5

Veggie Turkey Smash

Preparation Time: 15 Minutes Cooking Time: 7 Hours Servings: 4
Ingredients:
- One eggplant
- One onion
- 9 oz ground turkey

Directions:
- One green pepper, chopped
- One tablespoon butter
- One teaspoon chili flake

1. Peel the eggplant and onion and chop both into small pieces.
2. Then combine the chopped vegetables with the green pepper.
3. Add butter, chili flakes, and ground turkey.
4. Mix and transfer to the slow cooker.
5. Cook the turkey smash for 7 hours on Low.
6. When the time is done, stir the cooked meal carefully and transfer to serving bowls. Enjoy!

Nutrition: Calories 196, Fat 10.2, Fiber 5.2, Carbs 10.7, Protein 19.2

Paprika Shrimp

Preparation Time: 10 Minutes Cooking Time: 60 Minutes Servings: 6
Ingredients:
- 1-pound shrimp, peeled
- ¼ teaspoon ground black pepper
- One teaspoon paprika

Directions:
- ¼ teaspoon minced garlic
- ¾ cup chicken stock

1. Sprinkle the peeled shrimp with the ground black pepper and paprika.
2. Then sprinkle the shrimp with the minced garlic and stir well.
3. Place the chicken stock in the slow cooker.

4. Add the seasoned shrimp and close the lid.
5. Cook the shrimp for 1 hour on High.
6. Then transfer the shrimps to the serving plate and serve!
Nutrition: Calories 92, Fat 1.4, Fiber 0.2, Carbs 1.5, Protein 17.4

Breakfast Pizza

Preparation Time: 15 Minutes Cooking Time: 3 Hours Servings: 4
Ingredients:
- Four tablespoons almond flour
- ½ teaspoon baking powder
- ¾ teaspoon salt
- Two eggs, beaten

Directions:
1. Mix the almond flour and baking powder.
- 4 oz ham, chopped
- One teaspoon Italian seasoning
- One teaspoon olive oil
- 3 oz Parmesan, grated

2. Add salt and beaten eggs and knead the dough. Reel out the dough by means of a rolling pin. Spray the slow cooker bowl with the olive oil. Place the rolled-out dough in the slow cooker.
3. Sprinkle the dough with the chopped ham and grated Parmesan.
4. Then sprinkle the pizza with the Italian seasoning. Close the lid and cook the pizza for 3 hours on High.
5. Then let the cooked pizza cool slightly and serve it!
Nutrition: Calories 320, Fat 24.7, Fiber 3.4, Carbs 8.5, Protein 20.3

Breakfast Sweet Pepper Hash

Preparation Time: 15 Minutes Cooking Time: 4 Hours
Servings: 4
Ingredients:
- 8 oz ground pork
- One onion, chopped
- Two sweet peppers, chopped
- One teaspoon ghee

Directions:
1. Mix the chopped onion and sweet pepper.
2. Add chickens' stock and ghee.
- ¼ cup chicken stock
- ½ teaspoon chili flakes
- 4 oz Cheddar cheese

3. Add the chili flakes and transfer the mix to the slow cooker.
4. Shred the cheddar cheese and add it to the slow cooker as well.
5. Add ground pork and stir the ingredients carefully with a spatula.
6. Close the lid and cook the hash for 4 hours on High.
7. Stir the meal and serve!
Nutrition: Calories 235, Fat 12.7, Fiber 1.4, Carbs 7.5, Protein 22.8

Pork Breakfast Sausages

Preparation Time: 15 Minutes Cooking Time: 7 Hours Servings: 3
Ingredients:
- 9 oz ground pork
- 1 oz onion, grated
- One tablespoon almond flour

- One teaspoon coconut flour

Directions:
1. Mix up together the ground pork and grated onion.
2. Add almond flour and coconut flour.
3. Then add ground black pepper and chili flakes.
4. Stir the mixture well and form small sausages.
- ¼ teaspoon ground black pepper
- ¾ teaspoon chili flakes
- One teaspoon ghee

5. Place the sausages in the slow cooker and add the ghee.
6. Cook the sausages for 7 hours on Low.
7. When the sausages are prepared, let them cool slightly.
8. Enjoy!

Nutrition: Calories 188, Fat 9.8, Fiber 2.9, Carbs 5.7, Protein 25.1

Potato Breakfast Mix

Preparation Time: 10 Minutes Cooking Time: 5 Hours Servings: 4
Ingredients:
- One tablespoon olive oil
- One garlic clove, minced
- Two big sweet potatoes, chopped
- One yellow onion, chopped
- 3 cups tomato juice

Directions:
- 4 ounces green chilies chopped
- 2 cups veggie stock
- One teaspoon allspice, ground
- A pinch of salt and black pepper
- Two teaspoons ginger, grated

1. In your slow cooker, mix the oil with the garlic, sweet potatoes, tomato juice, green chilies, stock, allspice, salt, pepper, ginger, toss, cover, and cook on Low for 5 hours.
2. Stir the mix again, divide between plates and serve for breakfast.
3. Enjoy!

Nutrition: Calories 203, Fat 3, Fiber 3, Carbs 16, Protein 8

Breakfast Veggie Casserole

Preparation Time: 10 Minutes Cooking Time: 5 Hours
Servings: 4
Ingredients:
- One yellow onion, chopped
- One tablespoon olive oil
- Three garlic cloves, minced
- One teaspoon smoked paprika
- ½ teaspoon cumin, ground
- Three carrots, sliced
- One tablespoon thyme, dried
- Two celery stalks, chopped

Directions:
- One red bell pepper, chopped
- One yellow bell pepper, chopped
- 12 ounces canned tomatoes, chopped
- 5 ounces veggie stock

- Two eggplants, chopped
- Two thyme sprigs
- A pinch of salt and black pepper

1. Grease your slow cooker with the oil, add onion, garlic, paprika, cumin, carrots, thyme, celery, red and yellow bell pepper, tomatoes, stock, thyme, salt, pepper, and top with eggplant slices. Cover, cook on Low for 5 hours, divide between plates and serve for breakfast.
2. Enjoy!

Nutrition: Calories 200, Fat 2, Fiber 1, Carbs 5, Protein 10

Cheddar Jalapeno Breakfast Sausages

Preparation Time: 5 Minutes Cooking Time: 6 Hours Servings: 12
Ingredients:
- 12 medium-sized breakfast sausages
- One jalapeno pepper, chopped
- ½ cup cheddar cheese, grated

Directions:
- ¼ cup heavy cream
- Salt and pepper to taste

1. Mix all items in a bowl, then put it into the slow cooker.
2. Set to cook on Low for 6 hours or on high for 4 hours.
3. Garnish with parsley on top.

Nutrition: Calories: 472 Carbohydrates: 1.2 Protein: 32.6 Fat: 42.4 Sugar: 0 Fiber: 0.4

Breakfast Veggie Salad

Preparation Time: 10 Minutes Cooking Time: 5 Hours Servings: 4
Ingredients:
- Six tomatoes halved
- Two red onions cut into quarters
- Four long red peppers, cut into strips
- Two yellow peppers, cut into wedges
- Six garlic cloves

Directions:
- One tablespoon baby caper, drained
- One teaspoon sweet paprika
- A pinch of salt and black pepper
- Four tablespoons olive oil
- Juice of ½ lemon

1. Add the oil to your slow cooker, add tomatoes, onions, long peppers, yellow peppers, garlic, capers, paprika, salt, pepper, lemon juice, toss, cover, and cook low for 5 hours.
2. Divide into bowls and serve for breakfast.
3. Enjoy!

Nutrition: Calories 189, Fat 3, Fiber 4, Carbs 14, Protein 7

Breakfast Pork and Avocado Mix

Preparation Time: 10 Minutes Cooking Time: 10 Hours Servings: 4
Ingredients:
- 4 pounds pork butt roast
- One tablespoon cumin powder
- Two tablespoons chili powder
- One teaspoon coriander, ground

Directions:
- One tablespoon oregano, dried

- Two yellow onions, sliced
- Two avocados, peeled, pitted, and sliced

1. In your slow cooker, mix pork butt with chili, cumin, oregano, coriander, and onions, toss, cover, and cook on Low for 10 hours. Shred meat, divide between plates, top with avocado slices, and serve for breakfast.Enjoy!

Nutrition: Calories 270, Fat 4, Fiber 10, Carbs 8, Protein 25

Eggplant Pate with Breadcrumbs

Preparation Time: 27 Minutes Cooking Time: 6 Hours Servings: 15
Ingredients:
- 5 medium eggplants
- 2 sweet green pepper
- 1 cup bread crumbs
- 1 teaspoon salt
- 1 tablespoon sugar
- ½ cup tomato paste

Directions:
1. Peel the eggplants and chop them.
- 2 yellow onion
- 1 tablespoon minced garlic
- ¼ chili pepper
- 1 teaspoon olive oil
- 1 teaspoon kosher salt
- 1 tablespoon mayonnaise

2. Sprinkle the chopped eggplants with the salt and let sit for 10 minutes.
3. Meanwhile, combine the tomato paste with the kosher salt and sugar.
4. Add minced garlic and mayonnaise. Whisk carefully. Then, peel the onions and chop.
5. Spray the slow cooker bowl with the olive oil. Add the chopped onions.
6. Strain the chopped eggplants to get rid of the eggplant juice and transfer the strained eggplants into the slow cooker bowl. After this, add the tomato paste mixture.
7. Chop the chili pepper and sweet green peppers and add them to the slow cooker too. Stir the mixture inside the slow cooker carefully and close the lid.
8. Cook the dish for 6 hours on LOW. When the time is done, transfer the prepared mix into a bowl and blend it until smooth with the hand blender's help.
9. Sprinkle the prepared plate with the bread crumbs. Enjoy!

Nutrition: Calories 83, Fat 1, Carbs 14, Protein 18

Red Beans with the Sweet Peas

Preparation Time: 21 Minutes Cooking Time: 6 Hours
Servings: 5
Ingredients:
- 1 cup red beans, dried
- 3 chicken stock
- 3 tablespoon tomato paste
- 1 onion - 1 teaspoon salt

Directions:
1. Soak the red beans in water for 8 hours in advance.
- 1 chili pepper
- 1 teaspoon sriracha - 1 tablespoon butter
- 1 teaspoon turmeric
- 1 cup green peas

2. After this, strain the red beans and put them in the slow cooker.

3. Add the chicken stock, salt, and turmeric. Close the slow cooker lid and cook the red beans for 4 hours on HIGH.
4. Meanwhile, peel the onion and slice it. Combine the sliced onion with the tomato paste, sriracha, and butter. Chop the chili pepper and add it to the onion mixture.
5. When the time is done, open the slow cooker lid and add the onion mixture.
6. Stir it very carefully and close the slow cooker lid. Cook the dish for 1 hour more on Low.
7. Stir the red beans mixture carefully again and add the green peas. Cook the dish on LOW for one more hour. After this, stir the dish gently and serve. Enjoy!
Nutrition: Calories 190, Fat 3, Carbs 18, Protein 11

Nutritious Burrito Bowl

Preparation Time: 18 Minutes Cooking Time: 7 Hours Servings: 6
Ingredients:
- 10 oz. chicken breast
- 1 tablespoon chili flakes
- 1 teaspoon salt
- 1 teaspoon onion powder
- 1 teaspoon minced garlic

Directions:
- ½ cup white beans, canned
- ¼ cup green peas - 1 cup chicken stock
- ½ avocado pitted
- 1 teaspoon ground black pepper

1. Put the chicken breast in the slow cooker. Sprinkle the chicken breast with the chili flakes, salt, onion powder, minced garlic, and ground black pepper. Add the chicken stock. Close the slow cooker lid and cook the dish for 2 hours on HIGH. After this, open the slow cooker lid and add the white beans and green peas. Mix and close the lid. Cook the dish for 5 hours more on LOW.
2. When the time is done, remove the meat, white beans, and green peas from the slow cooker. Transfer the white beans and green peas to the serving bowls. Shred the chicken breast and add it to the serving bowls too. After this, peel the avocado and chop it. Sprinkle the prepared burrito bowls with the chopped avocado. Enjoy!
Nutrition: Calories 192, Fat 7, Carbs 13, Protein 11

Quinoa Curry

Preparation Time: 20 Minutes Cooking Time: 9 Hours Servings: 7
Ingredients:
- 8 oz. potato
- 7 oz. cauliflower
- 1 cup onion, chopped
- 7 oz. chickpea, canned
- 1 cup tomatoes, chopped
- 13 oz. almond milk

Directions:
1. Peel the potatoes and chop them.
- 3 cup chicken stock
- 8 tablespoon quinoas
- 1/3 tablespoon miso
- 1 teaspoon minced garlic
- 2 teaspoon curry paste

2. Put the chopped potatoes, onion, and tomatoes into the slow cooker. Combine the miso, chicken stock, and curry paste.
3. Whisk the mixture until the ingredients are dissolved in the chicken stock. Pour the chicken stock in the slow cooker too. Separate the cauliflower into the florets.

4. Add the cauliflower florets and the chickpeas to the slow cooker.
5. Add the almond milk, quinoa, and minced garlic.
6. Close the slow cooker lid and cook the dish on LOW for 9 hours.
7. When the dish is cooked, chill it and then mix it gently.
8. Transfer the prepared curry quinoa to the bowls. Enjoy!
Nutrition: Calories 262, Fat 4, Carbs 18, Protein 12

Ham Pitta Pockets

Preparation Time: 14 Minutes Cooking Time: 1 Hour and 30 Minutes Servings: 6
Ingredients:
- 6 pita bread, sliced
- 7 oz. mozzarella, sliced
- 1 teaspoon minced garlic
- 7 oz. ham, sliced

Directions:
1. Preheat the slow cooker on HIGH for 30 minutes.
2. Combine the mayo, heavy cream, and minced garlic.
- 1 big tomato, sliced
- 1 tablespoon mayo
- 1 tablespoon heavy cream
3. Spread the inside of the pita bread with the mayo mixture.
4. After this, fill the pita bread with the sliced mozzarella, tomato, and ham.
5. Wrap the pita bread in foil and place them in the slow cooker.
6. Close the slow cooker lid and cook the dish for 1.5 hours on HIGH.
7. Then discard the foil and serve the prepared pita pockets immediately. Enjoy!
Nutrition: Calories 273, Fat 3, Carbs 10, Protein 10

Breakfast Meatloaf

Preparation Time: 18 Minutes Cooking Time: 7 Hours Servings: 8
Ingredients:
- 12 oz. ground beef
- 1 teaspoon salt
- 1 teaspoon ground coriander
- 1 tablespoon ground mustard
- ¼ teaspoon ground chili pepper

Directions:
1. Chop the white bread and combine it with the milk.
2. Stir, then set aside for 3 minutes.
- 6 oz. white bread
- ½ cup milk
- 1 teaspoon ground black pepper
- 3 tablespoon tomato sauce
3. Meanwhile, combine the ground beef, salt, ground coriander, ground mustard, ground chili pepper, and ground black pepper.
4. Stir the white bread mixture carefully and add it to the ground beef. Cover the bottom of the slow cooker bowl with foil.
5. Shape the meatloaf, place the uncooked meatloaf in the slow cooker, and then spread it with the tomato sauce. Close the slow cooker lid and cook the meatloaf for 7 hours on LOW.
6. Slice the prepared meatloaf and serve. Enjoy!
Nutrition: Calories 214, Fat 14, Carbs 12, Protein 9

Breakfast Sweet Pepper Rounds

Preparation Time: 10 Minutes Cooking Time: 3 Hours
Servings: 4
Ingredients:
- 2 red sweet pepper
- 7 oz. ground chicken
- 5 oz. Parmesan
- 1 tablespoon sour cream
- 1 tablespoon flour

Directions:
- 1 egg
- 2 teaspoon almond milk
- 1 teaspoon salt
- ½ teaspoon ground black pepper
- ¼ teaspoon butter

1. Combine the sour cream with the ground chicken, flour, ground black pepper, almond milk, and butter. Beat eggs into the mixture.
2. Remove the seeds from the sweet peppers and slice them roughly.
3. Place the pepper slices in the slow cooker and fill them with the ground chicken mixture.
4. After this, chop Parmesan into the cubes and add them to the sliced peppers.
5. Close the slow cooker lid and cook the dish for 3 hours on HIGH.
6. When the time is done, make sure that the ground chicken is cooked and the cheese is melted. Enjoy the dish immediately.

Nutrition: Calories 261, Fat 8, Carbs 13, Protein 21

Breakfast Cauliflower Hash

Preparation Time: 17 Minutes Cooking Time: 8 Hours
Servings: 5
Ingredients:
- 7 eggs - ¼ cup milk
- 1 teaspoon salt
- 1 teaspoon ground black pepper
- ½ teaspoon ground mustard
- 10 oz. cauliflower

Directions:
- ¼ teaspoon chili flakes
- 5 oz. breakfast sausages, chopped
- ½ onion, chopped
- 5 oz. Cheddar cheese, shredded

1. Wash the cauliflower carefully and separate it into the florets.
2. After this, shred the cauliflower florets. Put the eggs in a bowl, then whisk. Add the milk, salt, ground black pepper, ground mustard, chili flakes, and chopped onion into the whisked egg mixture. Put the shredded cauliflower in the slow cooker.
3. Add the whisked egg mixture. Add the shredded cheese and chopped sausages.
4. Stir the mixture gently and close the slow cooker lid.
5. Cook the dish on LOW for 8 hours. When the cauliflower hash is cooked, remove it from the slow cooker and mix up. Enjoy!

Nutrition: Calories 329, Fat 16, Carbs 10, Protein 23

Healthy Low Carb Walnut Zucchini Bread

Preparation Time: 17 Minutes Cooking Time: 3 Hours and 10 Minutes Servings: 12
Ingredients:
- 3 eggs
- 1/2 cup walnuts, chopped

- 2 cups zucchini, shredded
- 2 tsp vanilla
- 1/2 cup pure all-purpose sweetener
- 1/3 cup coconut oil, softened

Directions:
- 1/2 tsp baking soda
- 1 1/2 Tsp baking powder
- 2 tsp cinnamon
- 1/3 cup coconut flour
- 1 cup almond flour
- 1/2 Tsp salt

1. In a bowl, combine almond flour, baking soda, baking powder, cinnamon, coconut flour, and salt. Set aside. In another bowl, whisk together eggs, vanilla, sweetener, and oil.
2. Add dry mixture to the wet mixture and fold well.
3. Add walnut and zucchini and fold well. Pour batter into the silicone bread pan.
4. Place the bread pan into the slow cooker on the rack.
5. Cover slow cooker with lid and cook on high for 3 hours.
6. Cut bread loaf into slices and serve.

Nutrition: Calories 174, Fat 15, Carbs 5, Protein 7

Bacon & Cheese Frittata

Preparation Time: 15 Minutes Cooking Time: 2 Hours and 30 Minutes Servings: 8

Ingredients:
- 1/2 lb. bacon
- 2 tablespoons butter
- 8 oz fresh spinach, packed down - 10 eggs

Directions:
1. Butter or grease the inside of your slow-cooker.
2. Loosely chop the spinach.
3. Cut bacon into half-inch pieces.
- 1/2 cup heavy whipping cream
- 1/2 cup shredded cheese
- Salt and pepper

4. Beat the eggs with the spices, cream, cheese, and chopped spinach. Then everything will be blended smoothly.
5. Line the bottommost of the slow cooker with the bacon.
6. Pour the egg mixture over the bacon.
7. Cover the slow cooker and adjust the temperature to high
8. Cook for 2 hours. Serve hot.

Nutrition: Calories 392, Fat 34, Carbs 4, Protein 19

Low-Carb Hash Brown Breakfast Casserole

Preparation Time: 10 Minutes Cooking Time: 6 Hours Servings: 6

Ingredients:
- 1 tablespoon unsalted butter, Ghee, or extra-virgin olive oil
- 12 large eggs
- ½ cup heavy (whipping) cream
- ½ teaspoon ground mustard

Directions:
- 1 head cauliflower, shredded or minced
- 1 onion, diced
- 10 ounces cooked breakfast sausage links, sliced
- 2 cups shredded Cheddar cheese, divided

1. Generously coat the inside part of the slow cooker insert with the butter.

2. In a large bowl, beat the eggs, whisk in heavy cream, one teaspoon of salt, ½ teaspoon of pepper, and the ground mustard.
3. Spread about one-third of the cauliflower in an even layer in the bottom of the cooker.
4. Layer one-third of the onions over the cauliflower, then one-third of the sausage, and top with ½ cup of Cheddar cheese. Season with salt and pepper. Repeat twice more with the remaining ingredients. You should have ½ cup of Cheddar cheese left.
5. Pour the egg mixture evenly over the layered ingredients, then sprinkle the remaining ½ cup Cheddar cheese on top. Cover then cook for 6 hours on low. Serve hot.
Nutrition: Calories 523, Fat 18, Carbs 7, Protein 3

Asparagus Smoked Salmon

Preparation Time: 15 Minutes Cooking Time: 5 Hours
Servings: 6
Ingredients:
- 1 tablespoon extra-virgin olive oil
- 6 large eggs
- 1 cup heavy (whipping) cream
- 2 teaspoons chopped fresh dill, plus additional for garnish
- ½ teaspoon kosher salt

Directions:
- ¼ teaspoon freshly ground black pepper
- 1½ cups shredded Havarti or Monterey Jack cheese
- 12 ounces asparagus, trimmed and sliced
- 6 ounces smoked salmon, flaked

1. Generously coat the inside part of the slow cooker insert with the olive oil.
2. In a large bowl, beat the eggs, then whisk in the heavy cream, dill, salt, and pepper.
3. Stir in the cheese and asparagus.
4. Gently fold in the salmon and then pour the mixture into the prepared insert.
5. Put the lid and cook for 6 hours on low or 3 hours on high.
6. Serve warm, garnished with additional fresh dill.
Nutrition: Calories 388, Fat 19, Carbs 10, Protein 21

Onion Broccoli Quiche

Preparation Time: 10 Minutes Cooking Time: 2 Hours and 30 Minutes Servings: 8
Ingredients:
- 9 eggs
- 2 cups cheese, shredded and divided
- 8 oz cream cheese
- 1/4 Tsp onion powder

Directions:
- 3 cups broccoli, cut into florets
- 1/4 Tsp pepper
- 3/4 Tsp salt

1. Add broccoli into the boiling water and cook for 3 minutes. Drain well and set aside to cool.
2. Add eggs, cream cheese, onion powder, pepper, and salt in mixing bowl and beat until well combined. Spray slow cooker from inside using cooking spray.
3. Add cooked broccoli into the slow cooker, then sprinkle half cup cheese. Pour egg mixture over broccoli and cheese mixture.
4. Cover slow cooker and cook on high for 2 hours and 15 minutes.
5. Once it is done, then sprinkle the remaining cheese and cover for 10 minutes or until cheese melted. Serve warm and enjoy.
Nutrition: Calories 296, Fat 24, Carbs 3, Protein 16

Thyme Sausage Squash

Preparation Time: 15 Minutes Cooking Time: 6 Hours Servings: 4
Ingredients:
- 2 tablespoons extra-virgin olive oil
- 14 ounces smoked chicken sausage, halved lengthwise and thinly sliced crosswise
- ¼ cup chicken broth
- 1 onion, halved and sliced
- ½ medium butternut squash, peeled, seeds and pulp removed and diced
- 1 small green bell pepper, seeded plus sliced into 1-inch-wide strips
- ½ small red bell pepper, seeded and sliced into 1-inch-wide strips
- ½ small yellow bell pepper, seeded and sliced into 1-inch-wide strips
- ½ teaspoon freshly ground black pepper
- 1 cup shredded Swiss cheese

Directions:
1. Combine all the ingredients. Cover and cook for 6 hours on low.
2. Just before serving, sprinkle the Swiss cheese over the top, cover, and cook for about 3 minutes more to melt the cheese.
3. Omit the cheese, and use a paleo-friendly sausage or diced ham.

Nutrition: Calories 502, Fat 26, Carbs 13, Protein 27

Tasty Greek Style Breakfast

Preparation Time: 10 Minutes Cooking Time: 5 Hours and 20 Minutes Servings: 6
Ingredients:
- 8 oz spinach
- 3 cloves chopped garlic
- 12 eggs
- 1/2 cup milk

Directions:
1. Butter or grease the inside of your slow cooker.
- 8 oz sliced crimini mushrooms
- 4 oz sun-dried tomatoes
- 1 cup feta cheese
- Salt and pepper

2. Beat together the eggs, milk, garlic, salt, and pepper separately from the other ingredients.
3. Put in the sun-dried tomatoes, sliced mushrooms, and spinach, stirring well.
4. Put the egg mixture in the slow-cooker.
5. Top it off with the feta cheese. Cover the slow cooker and set it on the low setting. Cook for five hours. Serve hot and enjoy!

Nutrition: Calories 236, Fat 15, Carbs 7, Protein 18

CHAPTER 2: LUNCH

Lime Chicken with Savoy Cabbage

Preparation Time: 10 Minutes Cooking Time: 7 Hours Servings: 4
Ingredients:
- 8 chicken thighs, skinless
- 2 cups Savoy cabbage, chopped
- 1 stalk celery, diced
- 1 medium onion, diced
- 1 tbsp ginger, grated
- ½ cup chicken stock

Directions:
- 2 limes
- 1 tsp salt
- 1 tsp black pepper
- Extra virgin olive oil
- Spicy squash noodles for serving

1. Place 4 tbsp extra virgin olive oil in the slow cooker, spread around the bottom. Add the ginger and onions.
2. Slice lime into ½" thick circles.
3. Place chicken in bottom of the slow cooker, and sprinkle with ½ tsp salt and ½ tsp black pepper.
4. Top with lime slices. On top of those, place celery and cabbage.
5. Pour in chicken stock, and cook on low for 7 hours.
6. Serve with Spicy Squash Noodles.

Nutrition: Calories 273, Carbs 5.7 g, Fat 12 g, Protein 34 g, Sodium 689 mg, Sugar 0 g

Middle Eastern Lamb Zucchini Casserole

Preparation Time: 20 Minutes Cooking Time: 7 Hours Servings: 6
Ingredients:
- 4 zucchinis, peeled
- 1 lb. ground lamb
- ½ cup coconut cream
- 2 eggs
- ¼ cup Parmesan
- ½ tsp cinnamon

Directions:
1. Using a mandolin, thinly-slice zucchini lengthwise.
- ½ tsp cloves
- ½ tsp cumin
- 1 tsp salt
- 1 tsp black pepper
- Extra virgin olive oil

2. Heat 3 tbsp extra virgin olive oil in a skillet. Add lamb, cinnamon, cloves, and cumin. Brown.
3. Combine coconut cream with egg, salt, and black pepper.
4. Coat slow cooker with olive oil, place ¼ of zucchini strips on the bottom of the slow cooker.
5. Next, brush coconut cream mixture on zucchini.
6. Place another layer of zucchini and half the remaining coconut cream, top with lamb, another layer of zucchini, remaining coconut cream.
7. Cook on low for 7 hours.

Nutrition: Calories 203, Carbs 4.7 g, Fat 10 g, Protein 25 g, Sodium 479 mg, Sugar 0 g

Ginger Steak Broccoli

Preparation Time: 10 Minutes Cooking Time: 4 Hours Servings: 4

Ingredients:
- 1 lb. sirloin steak
- 3 cups broccoli florets (frozen ok)
- 1 cup low-sodium beef stock
- 1 tbsp grated ginger

Directions:
- ½ tsp thyme
- 1 tsp salt
- 1 tsp black pepper
- Extra virgin olive oil

1. Slice sirloin steak against the grain into ½" wide strips.
2. Place 4 tbsp extra virgin olive oil in a skillet, add steak, and brown for a minute on each side.
3. Place steak, broccoli florets, along with ginger, beef stock, and soy sauce in the slow cooker.
4. Cook on medium-high for 4 hours.
5. Enjoy alone or with cauliflower rice.

Nutrition: Calories 273, Carbs 6 g, Fat 11 g, Protein 37 g, Sodium 714 mg, Sugar 0 g

BLT Chicken Salad

Preparation Time: 20 Minutes **Cooking Time:** 4 Hours **Servings:** 4

Ingredients:
- 4 x 4oz chicken breast
- 2 cup low-sodium chicken broth
- 8 slices bacon
- 2 cups romaine lettuce
- 1 tomato, diced

Directions:
- 1 tsp salt
- 1 tsp black pepper
- ¼ cup organic mayonnaise
- Extra virgin olive oil

1. Coat slow cooker with a little olive oil, and set on high.
2. Tenderize chicken breast, and sprinkle each chicken breast with salt and black pepper.
3. Wrap each chicken breast with bacon, and place it in a slow cooker.
4. Cook chicken breast on high for 4 hours.
5. Place mayonnaise with 1 tsp black pepper and 4 tbsp extra virgin olive oil in a blender. Mix until smooth.
6. Combine lettuce, tomato in a bowl, and toss with mayo dressing.
7. Top salad with chicken breast and serve.

Nutrition: Calories 366, Carbs 6 g, Fat 19 g, Protein 43 g, Sodium 1183 mg, Sugar 0 g

Figs and Goat Cheese-Stuffed Chicken

Preparation Time: 20 Minutes **Cooking Time:** 8 Hours **Servings:** 4

Ingredients:
- 4 x 4oz chicken breasts
- 4 figs
- ½ cup goat cheese, crumbled

Directions:
- 1 tsp salt
- 1 tsp black pepper
- Extra virgin olive oil

1. Combine 3 tbsp olive oil, salt, black pepper in a bowl, and rub onto chicken breasts. Marinate for an hour.
2. Remove fig skin, and slice figs into ½" pieces. Combine with goat cheese.
3. Turn slow cooker to low.
4. Place plastic wrap over chicken breasts and pound with a mallet until each breast is approximately

¼" thick (or ask your butcher to do it).
5. Scoop a quarter of the cheese-fig mixture into the chicken, roll up chicken breast, and place in the slow cooker. Repeat for each chicken breast.
6. Cook on low for 8 hours.
7. Serve with a green salad.
Nutrition: Calories 369, Carbs 7 g, Fat 18 g, Protein 46 g, Sodium 811 mg, Sugar 0 g

Carne Asada

Preparation Time: 10 Minutes Cooking Time: 8 Hours Servings: 8
Ingredients:
- 4 lb. chuck roast
- 1 onion, chopped
- 4 limes, juiced
- ½ cup cilantro, minced
- 8 cloves garlic, minced

Directions:
1. Rinse pot roast and pat dry.
- 2 tsp paprika
- 2 tsp oregano
- 2 tsp cumin
- 2 tsp salt
- 1 tsp black pepper

2. Combine remaining ingredients in a blender, and mix until well combined.
3. Brush slow cooker with extra virgin olive oil, and set on high.
4. Coat pot roast with cilantro topping.
5. Place in the slow cooker, and cook for 8 hours.
6. Serve with Cauliflower Rice.
Nutrition: Calories 506, Carbs 3 g, Fat 19g, Protein 75 g, Sodium 733 mg, Sugar 0 g

Amazing Pulled Pork

Preparation Time: 25 Minutes Cooking Time: 8 Hours Servings: 8
Ingredients:
- 5 lb. pork shoulder
- 2 tbsp mustard
- 2 cups tomato purée
- 6 Medjool Dates, pitted
- ½ tsp cloves, ground
- ½ tsp cinnamon
- 2 tsp salt

Directions:
- Extra virgin olive oil Tortilla Wraps
- 8 eggs
- 1 tbsp coconut flour
- ½ tsp salt

1. Place pitted dates in a blender, and mix until paste forms, add tomato purée, cinnamon, salt, black pepper, and mix.
2. Combine mustard, blended tomato puree, cloves, cinnamon, salt, and mix.
3. Place pork shoulder in the slow cooker, pour the sauce into the slow cooker, and coat pork shoulder.
4. Cook pork for 8 hours on high. Once the pork is cooked, use a fork to shred.
5. For tortilla wraps, whisk eggs, add milk and flour, and mix until well combined.
6. Heat 4 tbsp oil in a skillet on medium-high.
7. Pour 1/8th of the mixture into skillet and cook each side 30 seconds.

8. Spoon pork mixture into egg tortilla and serve.
Nutrition: Calories 777, Carbs 8 g, Fat 55 g, Protein 59 g, Sodium 835 mg, Sugar 5 g

Braised Pork Belly

Preparation Time: 10 Minutes Cooking Time: 4 Hours Servings: 8
Ingredients:
- 1 lb. pork belly
- 2 medium onions, diced
- 1 tsp Dijon mustard

Directions:
- ½ cup apple sauce
- 1 tsp black pepper
- 1 tsp salt

1. Heat extra virgin olive oil in the skillet, add onion, sauté for a minute.
2. Place onion in the slow cooker, add pork belly, apple sauce. Cook on high for 4 hours.
3. Serve with Walnut Cabbage Salad.

Nutrition: Calories 278, Carbs 3.5 g, Fat 15 g, Protein 26 g, Sodium 1214 mg, Sugar 0 g

Peppercorn Short Ribs

Preparation Time: 10 Minutes Cooking Time: 4 Hours Servings: 8
Ingredients:
- 4 lbs. short ribs, bone-in
- 8 peppercorns
- 2 cups low-sodium beef
- 1 onion, diced
- 2 carrots, peeled, diced
- 2 celery stalks, diced
- 4 cloves, minced

Directions:
- 1 tsp thyme
- 1 tsp rosemary
- 2 bay leaves
- 2 tsp salt
- 2 tsp black pepper
- Extra virgin olive oil

1. Heat the extra virgin olive oil in a skillet. Add onions and garlic, and sauté until brown.
2. Place the onion mixture in the slow cooker, add short ribs, carrots, celery stalk, cloves, thyme, rosemary, peppercorns, bay leaves, salt, and black pepper.
3. Cook on high for 4 hours.

Nutrition: Calories 520, Carbs 3.7 g, Fat 24 g, Protein 67 g, Sodium 923 mg, Sugar 0 g

Spicy Italian Sausage and Zucchini Noodles

Preparation Time: 20 Minutes Cooking Time: 4 Hours Servings: 6
Ingredients:
- 6 Spicy Italian pork sausages
- 1 onion, peeled and diced
- 2 cups low-sodium chicken stock
- 1 tomato, diced

Directions:
- 4 zucchinis, peeled
- 1 tsp oregano - 1 tsp salt
- 1 tsp black pepper
- Extra virgin olive oil

1. Coat slow cooker with a little extra virgin olive oil, and set to high. Slice sausage into ½" thick rounds, and place in the slow cooker.
2. Heat 3 tbsp extra virgin olive oil in a skillet, add onion and garlic, sauté for a minute, and add to slow cooker.
3. Add tomatoes, oregano, and a tsp of salt and black pepper and chicken stock, cover, and cook for 4 hours. Using Mandolin, slice zucchini vertically to create thin Zucchini Noodles.
4. Top zucchini noodles with Spicy Italian Sausage and serve.
Nutrition: Calories 254, Carbs 8.5 g, Fat 14 g, Protein 24 g, Sodium 1044 mg, Sugar 3 g

Meaty Cauliflower Lasagna

Preparation Time: 20 Minutes Cooking Time: 5 Hours
Servings: 8
Ingredients:
- 1 lb. ground beef
- 1 small cauliflower head
- 1 red onion, diced
- 4 cloves garlic, minced
- 2 cups crushed tomato
- 1 cup Mozzarella, shredded

Directions:
- 1 egg
- 1 tsp oregano
- 1 bay leaf
- 1 tsp black pepper
- 1 tsp salt
- Extra virgin olive oil

1. Brush slow cooker with olive oil, and set the slow cooker on medium high.
2. Separate cauliflower into florets, peel the outer layer of cauliflower stem and dice stem.
3. Place cauliflower in a food processor, and pulse into rice-like granules, crack an egg into cauliflower and mix along with ½ tsp of salt.
4. Place 3 tbsp olive oil in a skillet, add ground beef, brown, add crushed tomatoes, oregano, bay leaf, black pepper, and ½ tsp salt, mix.
5. Place ½ cauliflower mixture in the slow cooker, next layer 1/3 of the beef mixture and ½ of cheese, place remaining cauliflower on top. Spoon remaining sauce on top of the cauliflower, sprinkle with remaining cheese. Cook on medium high for 5 hours.
Nutrition: Calories 342, Carbs 8.2 g, Fat 14 g, Protein 45 g, Sodium 681 mg, Sugar 0 g

Chili Verde

Preparation Time: 10 Minutes Cooking Time: 7 Hours Servings: 8
Ingredients:
- 1½ lbs. pork shoulder
- ½ lb. sirloin, cubed
- 4 Anaheim chiles, stemmed
- 6 cloves garlic, minced
- ½ cup cilantro, chopped
- 2 onions, peeled and sliced

Directions:
- 2 tomatoes, chopped.
- 1 tbsp tomato paste
- 1 lime
- 1 tbsp cumin
- 1 tbsp oregano
- Extra virgin olive oil

1. Slice pork shoulder into ½" cubes, and set slow cooker to medium.

2. Heat the extra virgin olive oil in a skillet, add onions, Anaheim chilies, garlic, and sauté for 2 minutes.
3. Place skillet mixture into the slow cooker, add pork shoulder, sirloin, and stir.
4. Add tomatoes, cilantro, tomato paste, cumin, oregano, and salt to the pot.
5. Cover and cook for 7 hours.
6. Squeeze a little lime in each bowl when serving.
Nutrition: Calories 262, Carbs 6 g, Fat 16 g, Protein 23 g, Sodium 63 mg, Sugar 0 g

Tandoori Salmon with Fresh Cucumber Salad

Preparation Time: 10 Minutes Cooking Time: 3 Hours Servings: 8
Ingredients:
- 4 x 4oz Wild salmon fillets
- 2 tsp Tandoori spice
- 1 tsp salt
- 1 tsp black pepper
- 4 tbsp ghee Cucumber Salad **Directions:**
- 1 English cucumber
- 1 cup arugula
- ½ cup parsley
- ¼ cup lemon juice
- 2 tbsp extra virgin olive oil

1. Heat ghee in a skillet over medium heat along with tandoori spice for a minute.
2. Place salmon fillets in the slow cooker, skin side down, sprinkle with salt, black pepper, and pour Tandoori butter over salmon.
3. Cook on high for 3.5 hours.
4. While salmon is cooking, dice the cucumber and toss with arugula, parsley, lemon juice, and extra virgin olive oil.
5. Serve salmon with fresh cucumber salad.
Nutrition: Calories 413, Carbs 4 g, Fat 34 g, Protein 25 g, Sodium 645 mg, Sugar 0 g

CHAPTER 3: DINNER

Hungarian Mushroom Soup

Preparation Time: 5 Minutes
Cooking Time: 2 Hours and 45 Minutes Servings: 5
Ingredients:
- 1 cup of white mushrooms, sliced
- 3 cups of chicken broth
- 2 large onions, chopped
- 4 tbsp of butter
- 1 tbsp of smoked paprika

Directions:
- 1 tbsp of soy sauce
- 1 tsp of dried dill
- 1 cup coconut cream
- 1 tsp of lemon pepper
- A pinch of salt

1. Sauté the mushrooms plus the onions and the butter in a frying pan for a couple of minutes.
2. Add to the slow cooker and combine it with the rest of the fixings. Set to cook on high heat for 2 ½ hours.
3. Serve as it is or blends to form a semi-thick, creamy soup.

Nutrition: Calories: 286, Fat: 26g, Carbs: 9g, Protein: 6,3g.

Curried Cauliflower

Preparation Time: 5 Minutes
Cooking Time: 2 Hours and 40 Minutes Servings: 5
Ingredients:
- 2 cups of medium cauliflower florets
- 1/3 cup tomato paste
- 2 tbsp of olive oil
- 1 tsp of cumin

Directions:
- 1 tbsp of curry
- 1 clove of garlic
- Salt
- Pepper

1. Combine all the spices, then season the cauliflower florets, making sure everything is covered evenly.
2. In a small dish, whisk the tomato paste and mayo and spread over the cauliflower florets.
3. Set the slow cooker on high heat and cook the cauliflower for 2 ½ hours.

Nutrition: Calories: 170, Fat: 11g, Carbs: 6g, Protein: 6g.

Cheese Stuffed and Pesto Eggplants

Preparation Time: 5 Minutes Cooking Time: 3 Hours
Servings: 4
Ingredients:
- 1 large eggplant, thinly cut lengthwise
- 1 ½ cup full fat cottage cheese
- ½ cup cream cheese
- 1 egg, beaten
- 1 tbsp of basil pesto

Directions:

- ½ cup grated Parmesan cheese
- 1/3 cup tomato sauce (low in sugar)
- 1 drizzle of olive oil
- Salt
- Pepper

1. Combine in a bowl the soft cheeses, pesto, and eggs to make a spreadable filling.
2. Lightly season the eggplants with salt and pepper and distribute the filling to each eggplant cut. Secure with a toothpick.
3. Add to the slow cooker and add the tomato sauce on top. Cook on high heat for 2 ½ hours. Add the Parmesan cheese and cook for another 20 minutes prior to serving.

Nutrition: Calories: 122, Fat:9g, Carbs: 5g, Protein: 10g.

Creamy Vegan Broccoli Soup

Preparation Time: 5 Minutes Cooking Time: 3 Hours
Servings: 5
Ingredients:
- 2 cups of broccoli florets
- 1 cup of full-fat coconut cream
- 2 tbsp of olive oil or ghee

Directions:
- 4 cups of vegetable stock
- 1 tbsp of nutritional yeast

1. Combine all the liquid ingredients with the nutritional yeast and whisk.
2. Place the broccoli in the slow cooker, pour over the liquid mixture, and cook on low heat for 3 hours.
3. Remove from the slow cooker and serve as it is or blend to form a uniform, creamy soup.

Nutrition: Calories: 291, Fat: 25g, Carbs: 5g, Protein: 13g.

The Ultimate Bacon Meatloaf

Preparation Time: 5 Minutes Cooking Time: 1 Hour and 40 Minutes
Servings: 7 to 8
Ingredients:
- 1 pound of ground pork
- 6 slices of bacon
- 1 tbsp of mustard
- 1 tbsp of tomato paste
- 1 egg

Directions:
- ½ cup of shredded cheddar cheese
- 1 tsp of fresh thyme
- Salt
- Pepper
- Combine the ground pork with the mustard, tomato paste, egg, fresh thyme, salt, and pepper.
- Arrange the bacon widthwise (half will be sticking out) into a greased loaf of bread pan of 9X5 inches. Place half of the mixture in the loaf pan over the bacon. Sprinkle the cheese in the middle and add the rest of the ground pork mixture. Fold over the hanging bacon bits. Add to the slow cooker and set on high heat for 1 ½ hours.

Nutrition: Calories: 370g, Fat: 26g, Carbs: 5g, Protein: 25g.

Cheese and Mushroom Stuffed Chicken Rolls

Preparation Time: 5 Minutes Cooking Time: 1 Hour and 30 Minutes
Servings: 6
Ingredients:

- 2 skinless chicken breasts, cut lengthwise into 3 pieces each and pounded
- ½ cup of Monterey jack cheese
- 1 tbsp of Herbed butter
- 1 scallion, chopped
- 1 clove of garlic, chopped
- ½ cup of sliced mushrooms
- 1/3 white wine
- Salt
- Pepper

Directions:
1. Season the chicken breasts lightly with salt and pepper.
2. In a small frying pan, heat the butter and sauté the onions with the garlic and scallion for a couple of minutes. Add the wine and turn off the heat
3. Spoon the mushrooms over each chicken breast piece, add half of the cheese, and roll with each piece. Secure with a toothpick.
4. Add the chicken rolls to the slow cooker and cook on high heat for 1 ½ hours. Sprinkle with the remaining cheese on top during the last 20 minutes of cooking.

Nutrition: Calories: 312, Fat: 19g, Carbs: 4,8, Protein: 22g.

Tasty Short Ribs

Preparation Time: 5 Minutes
Cooking Time: 8 Hours and 30 Minutes Servings: 6-7
Ingredients:
- 2 ½ pounds of short beef ribs
- 2 tbsp of butter
- 1 large onion, roughly chopped
- 1 large carrot, roughly chopped,
- 1 celery stalk, chopped

Directions:
1. Combine the tomatoes, stock, and red wine together
- 1 cup of diced tomatoes
- ½ cup of red wine
- 1 tsp of dried rosemary
- 1 bay leaf
- 1 cup of vegetable stock

2. Place the ribs in the slow cooker and pour over the wine mixture.
3. Add the veggies on the sides.
4. Set to low heat and cook for 8 ½ hours.

Nutrition: Calories: 476, Fat: 18g, Carbs: 8g, Protein: 21g.

Garlic Butter Turkey Breasts

Preparation Time: 5 Minutes
Cooking Time: 3 Hours and 30 Minutes Servings: 4
Ingredients:
- 2 large turkey breasts (skin off)
- 2 tbsp of butter
- 2 cloves of garlic, minced
- 1/3 cup of chopped parsley

Directions:
- ½ cup white dry wine
- Salt
- Pepper

1. Combine the garlic with the melted butter and slather on the turkey breasts in the slow cooker. Season with salt and pepper and pour over the wine. Finish with the parsley on top.
2. Set your slow cooker and cook in low heat for 3 ½ hours.
Nutrition: Calories: 282, Fat: 19,2g. Carbs: 4g, Protein: 19g.

Creamy Salmon and Dill

Preparation Time: 15 Minutes Cooking Time: 2 Hours Servings: 4 to 5
Ingredients:
- 4 -5 medium skin-on salmon fillets
- 1 tsp of black peppercorns
- 2 cups of low sodium vegetable stock
- 1/3 cup white dry wine
-

Directions:
- 1 shallot, thinly sliced
- 1 tsp of lemon zest
- 1 tsp of Dill
- 1/3 cup of heavy cream

1. Combine all the ingredients in the slow cooker except the heavy cream.
2. Set on low heat and cook for 2 hours. Add in the heavy cream, whisk lightly, and cook for another 10 minutes on low heat.
Nutrition: Calories: 510, Fat: 35g, Carbs: 2g, Protein: 44g.

Shrimps Alfredo

Preparation Time: 5 Minutes Cooking Time: 1 Hour and 30 Minutes
Servings: 4 to 5
Ingredients:
- 1 pound of raw shrimps
- 4 oz. of cream cheese
- ½ cup of coconut cream
- 1 tbsp of butter
- ½ cup of Parmesan cheese

Directions:
- 1 tbsp of garlic powder
- 1 tbsp of basic
- Salt
- Pepper

1. Combine all the ingredients together in a bowl except the shrimps.
2. Add the shrimps to the slow cooker and pour over the cream cheese mixture.
3. Set on low heat for 1 ½ hour.
4. Serve optionally with cauliflower rice.
Nutrition: Calories: 298, Fat: 17g, Carbs: 7,2, Protein: 23g.

Mediterranean Fresh Tuna

Preparation Time: 5 Minutes Cooking Time: 2 Hours
Servings: 5
Ingredients:
- 4-5 fresh tuna steaks
- 1 tbsp of capers
- 2 tbsp of olive oil
- ¼ cup chopped black olives
- 1.2 cup of cubed tomatoes

Directions:
- 1 tsp of thyme
- 1/3 cup white dry wine
- Salt
- Pepper

1. Brush the tuna with the oil and season with thyme, salt, and pepper.
2. Add to the slow cooker with the rest of the ingredients evenly arranged on top.
3. Set on high heat and cook for 2 hours.

Nutrition: Calories: 372, Fat: 16g, Carbs: 3g, Protein: 40g.

Low Carb Seafood and Sausage Gumbo

Preparation Time: 5 Minutes Cooking Time: 1 Hour and 30 Minutes
Servings: 6
Ingredients:
- ½ cup of clarified butter
- ½ cup of scallions, chopped
- 2/3 cup celery, chopped
- 1 lb. of mixed seafood
- 1 large Italian sausage, crumbled

Directions:
1. Sauté lightly the sausages and the onions in butter.
- 1 tsp of low carb creole seasoning
- 1 large bay leave
- 6 cups of chicken broth
- ½ cup heavy cream

2. Combine with all the rest of the ingredients in the slow cooker and set to cook on high heat for 1 ½ hour (make sure you add the fresh cream towards the last minutes of cooking).

Nutrition: Calories: 343g. Fat: 27g, Carbs: 4g, Protein: 21g

CHAPTER 4: SIDE DISHES

Zucchini Pasta

Preparation Time: 15 Minutes Cooking Time: 60 Minutes Servings: 4
Ingredients:
- 2 zucchinis
- 1 teaspoon dried oregano
- 1 teaspoon dried basil

Directions:
- 2 tablespoons butter
- ¼ teaspoon salt
- 5 tablespoons water

1. Peel the zucchini and spiralize it with a veggie spiralizer.
2. Melt the butter and mix it together with the dried oregano, dried basil, salt, and water.
3. Place the spiralized zucchini in the slow cooker and add the spice mixture.
4. Close the lid and cook the meal for 1 hour on Low.
5. Let the cooked pasta cool slightly.
6. Serve it!

Nutrition: Calories 68, Fat 6, Fiber 1.2, Carbs 3.5, Protein 1.3

Chinese Broccoli

Preparation Time: 15 Minutes Cooking Time: 60 Minutes Servings: 4
Ingredients:
- 1 tablespoon sesame seeds
- 1 tablespoon olive oil
- 10 oz broccoli
- 1 teaspoon chili flakes

Directions:
- 1 tablespoon apple cider vinegar
- 3 tablespoons water
- ¼ teaspoon garlic powder

1. Cut the broccoli into the florets and sprinkle with the olive oil, chili flakes, apple cider vinegar, and garlic powder.
2. Stir the broccoli and place it in the slow cooker.
3. Add water and sesame seeds.
4. Cook the broccoli for 1 hour on High.
5. Transfer the cooked broccoli to serving plates and enjoy!

Nutrition: Calories 69, Fat 4.9, Fiber 2.1, Carbs 5.4, Protein 2.4

Slow Cooker Spaghetti Squash

Preparation Time: 15 Minutes Cooking Time: 4 Hours
Servings: 5
Ingredients:
- 1-pound spaghetti squash
- 1 tablespoon butter
- ¼ cup of water

Directions:
- 1 teaspoon ground black pepper
- ¼ teaspoon ground nutmeg

1. Peel the spaghetti squash and sprinkle it with the ground black pepper and ground nutmeg.
2. Pour water into the slow cooker.

3. Add butter and spaghetti squash.
4. Close the lid and cook for 4 hours on Low.
5. Chop the spaghetti squash into small pieces and serve!
Nutrition: Calories 50, Fat 2.9, Fiber 6.6, Carbs 0.1, Protein 0.7

Mushroom Stew

Preparation Time: 15 Minutes Cooking Time: 6 Hours Servings: 8
Ingredients:
- 10 oz white mushrooms, sliced
- 2 eggplants, chopped
- 1 onion, diced
- 1 garlic clove, diced
- 2 bell peppers, chopped

Directions:
- 1 cup of water
- 1 tablespoon butter
- ½ teaspoon salt
- ½ teaspoon ground black pepper

1. Place the sliced mushrooms, chopped eggplant, and diced onion into the slow cooker.
2. Add the garlic clove and bell peppers.
3. Sprinkle the vegetables with salt and ground black pepper.
4. Add butter and water and stir it gently with a wooden spatula.
5. Close the lid and cook the stew for 6 hours on Low.
6. Stir the cooked stew one more time and serve!
Nutrition: Calories 71, Fat 1.9, Fiber 5.9, Carbs 13, Protein 3

Cabbage Steaks

Preparation Time: 15 Minutes Cooking Time: 2 Hours Servings: 4
Ingredients:
- 10 oz white cabbage
- 1 tablespoon butter
- ½ teaspoon cayenne pepper

Directions:
- ½ teaspoon chili flakes
- 4 tablespoons water

1. Slice the cabbage into medium steaks and rub them with the cayenne pepper and chili flakes.
2. Rub the cabbage steaks with butter on each side.
3. Place them in the slow cooker and sprinkle with water.
4. Close the lid and cook the cabbage steaks for 2 hours on High.
5. When the cabbage steaks are cooked, they should be tender to the touch.
6. Serve the cabbage steak after 10 minutes of chilling.
Nutrition: Calories 44, Fat 3, Fiber 1.8, Carbs 4.3, Protein 1

Mashed Cauliflower

Preparation Time: 20 Minutes Cooking Time: 3 Hours Servings: 5
Ingredients:
- 3 tablespoons butter
- 1-pound cauliflower
- 1 tablespoon full-fat cream

Directions:
1. Wash the cauliflower and chop it.
2. Place the chopped cauliflower in the slow cooker.

3. Add butter and full-fat cream.
4. Add salt and ground black pepper.
5. Stir the mixture and close the lid.
6. Cook the cauliflower for 3 hours on High.
- 1 teaspoon salt
- 1 teaspoon ground black pepper
- 1 oz dill, chopped

7. When the cauliflower is cooked, transfer it to a blender and blend until smooth.
8. Place the smooth cauliflower in a bowl and mix it with the chopped dill.
9. Stir it well and serve!

Nutrition: Calories 101, Fat 7.4, Fiber 3.2, Carbs 8.3, Protein 3.1

Bacon-Wrapped Cauliflower

Preparation Time: 15 Minutes Cooking Time: 7 Hours
Servings: 4
Ingredients:
- 11 oz cauliflower head
- 3 oz bacon, sliced
- 1 teaspoon salt

Directions:
- 1 teaspoon cayenne pepper
- 1 oz butter, softened
- ¾ cup of water

1. Sprinkle the cauliflower head with the salt and cayenne pepper, then rub with butter.
2. Wrap the cauliflower head in the sliced bacon and secure with toothpicks.
3. Pour water into the slow cooker and add the wrapped cauliflower head.
4. Cook the cauliflower head for 7 hours on Low.
5. Then let the cooked cauliflower head cool for 10 minutes.
6. Serve it!

Nutrition: Calories 187, Fat 14.8, Fiber 2.1, Carbs 4.7, Protein 9.5

Cauliflower Casserole

Preparation Time: 15 Minutes Cooking Time: 7 Hours Servings: 5
Ingredients:
- 2 tomatoes, chopped
- 11 oz cauliflower chopped
- 5 oz broccoli, chopped
- 1 cup of water

Directions:
1. Mix the water, salt, and chili flakes.
2. Place the butter in the slow cooker.
3. Add a layer of the chopped cauliflower.
4. Add the layer of broccoli and tomatoes.
- 1 teaspoon salt
- 1 tablespoon butter
- 5 oz white mushrooms, chopped
- 1 teaspoon chili flakes

5. Add the mushrooms and pat down the mix to flatten.
6. Add the water and close the lid.
7. Cook the casserole for 7 hours on Low.
8. Cool the casserole to room temperature and serve!

Nutrition: Calories 61, Fat 2.6, Fiber 3.2, Carbs 8.1, Protein 3.4

Cauliflower Rice

Preparation Time: 15 Minutes Cooking Time: 2 Hours Servings: 5
Ingredients:
- 1-pound cauliflower
- 1 teaspoon salt
- 1 tablespoon turmeric

Directions:
- 1 tablespoon butter
- ¾ cup water

1. Chop the cauliflower into tiny pieces to make cauliflower rice. You can also pulse in a food processor to get very fine grains of 'rice'.
2. Place the cauliflower rice in the slow cooker.
3. Add salt, turmeric, and water.
4. Stir gently and close the lid.
5. Cook the cauliflower rice for 2 hours on High.
6. Strain the cauliflower rice and transfer it to a bowl.
7. Add butter and stir gently.
8. Serve it!

Nutrition: Calories 48, Fat 2.5, Fiber 2.6, Carbs 5.7, Protein 1.9

Curry Cauliflower

Preparation Time: 15 Minutes Cooking Time: 5 Hours Servings: 2
Ingredients:
- 10 oz cauliflower
- 1 teaspoon curry paste
- 1 teaspoon curry powder
- ½ teaspoon dried cilantro

Directions:
- 1 oz butter
- ¾ cup of water
- ¼ cup chicken stock

1. Chop the cauliflower roughly and sprinkle it with the curry powder and dried cilantro.
2. Place the chopped cauliflower in the slow cooker.
3. Mix the curry paste with the water.
4. Add chicken stock and transfer the liquid to the slow cooker.
5. Add butter and close the lid.
6. Cook the cauliflower for 5 hours on Low.
7. Strain ½ of the liquid off and discard. Transfer the cauliflower to serving bowls.
8. Serve it!

Nutrition: Calories 158, Fat 13.3, Fiber 3.9, Carbs 8.9, Protein 3.3

Garlic Cauliflower Steaks

Preparation Time: 15 Minutes Cooking Time: 3 Hours Servings: 4
Ingredients:
- 14 oz cauliflower head
- 1 teaspoon minced garlic
- 4 tablespoons butter

Directions:
- 4 tablespoons water
- 1 teaspoon paprika

1. Wash the cauliflower head carefully and slice it into the medium steaks.
2. Mix up together the butter, minced garlic, and paprika.

3. Rub the cauliflower steaks with the butter mixture.
4. Pour the water into the slow cooker.
5. Add the cauliflower steaks and close the lid.
6. Cook the vegetables for 3 hours on High.
7. Transfer the cooked cauliflower steaks to a platter and serve them immediately!
Nutrition: Calories 129, Fat 11.7, Fiber 2.7, Carbs 5.8, Protein 2.2

Zucchini Gratin

Preparation Time: 10 Minutes **Cooking Time:** 5 Hours **Servings:** 3
Ingredients:
- 1 zucchini, sliced
- 3 oz Parmesan, grated
- 1 teaspoon ground black pepper

Directions:
- 1 tablespoon butter
- ½ cup almond milk

1. Sprinkle the sliced zucchini with the ground black pepper.
2. Chop the butter and place it in the slow cooker.
3. Transfer the sliced zucchini to the slow cooker to make the bottom layer.
4. Add the almond milk.
5. Sprinkle the zucchini with the grated cheese and close the lid.
6. Cook the gratin for 5 hours on Low.
7. Then let the gratin cool until room temperature.
8. Serve it!
Nutrition: Calories 229, Fat 19.6, Fiber 1.8, Carbs 5.9, Protein 10.9

Eggplant Gratin

Preparation Time: 15 Minutes **Cooking Time:** 5 Hours **Servings:** 7
Ingredients:
- 1 tablespoon butter
- 1 teaspoon minced garlic
- 2 eggplants, chopped
- 1 teaspoon salt

Directions:
1. Mix the dried parsley, chili flakes, and salt.
- 1 tablespoon dried parsley
- 4 oz Parmesan, grated
- 4 tablespoons water
- 1 teaspoon chili flakes
2. Sprinkle the chopped eggplants with the spice mixture and stir well.
3. Place the eggplants in the slow cooker.
4. Add the water and minced garlic.
5. Add the butter and sprinkle with the grated Parmesan.
6. Close the lid and cook the gratin for 5 hours on Low.
7. Open the lid and cool the gratin for 10 minutes.
8. Serve it.
Nutrition: Calories 107, Fat 5.4, Fiber 5.6, Carbs 10, Protein 6.8

Moroccan Eggplant Mash

Preparation Time: 15 Minutes **Cooking Time:** 7 Hours **Servings:** 4
Ingredients:
- 1 eggplant, peeled

- 1 jalapeno pepper
- 1 teaspoon curry powder
- ½ teaspoon salt
- 1 teaspoon paprika

Directions:
1. Chop the eggplant into small pieces.
2. Place the eggplant in the slow cooker.
- ¾ teaspoon ground nutmeg
- 2 tablespoons butter
- ¾ cup almond milk
- 1 teaspoon dried dill
3. Chop the jalapeno pepper and combine it with the eggplant.
4. Then sprinkle the vegetables with the curry powder, salt, paprika, ground nutmeg, and dried dill.
5. Add almond milk and butter.
6. Close the lid and cook the vegetables for 7 hours on Low.
7. Cool the vegetables and then blend them until smooth with a hand blender.
8. Transfer the cooked eggplant mash into the bowls and serve!

Nutrition: Calories 190, Fat 17, Fiber 5.6, Carbs 10, Protein 2.5

Sautéed Bell Peppers

Preparation Time: 15 Minutes Cooking Time: 5 Hours Servings: 6
Ingredients:
- 8 oz bell peppers
- 7 oz cauliflower, chopped
- 2 oz bacon, chopped
- 1 teaspoon salt
- 1 teaspoon ground black pepper

Directions:
- ¾ cup coconut milk, unsweetened
- 1 teaspoon butter
- 1 teaspoon thyme
- 1 onion, diced
- 1 teaspoon turmeric

1. Remove the seeds from the bell peppers and chop them roughly.
2. Place the bell peppers, cauliflower, and bacon in the slow cooker.
3. Add the salt, ground black pepper, coconut milk, butter, milk, and thyme.
4. Stir well, then add the diced onion.
5. Add the turmeric and stir the mixture.
6. Close the lid and cook 5 hours on Low.
7. When the meal is cooked, let it chill for 10 minutes and serve it!

Nutrition: Calories 195, Fat 12.2, Fiber 4.2, Carbs 13.1, Protein 6.7

CHAPTER 5: SNACKS AND APPETIZERS

Chicken Bites

Preparation Time: 15 Minutes Cooking Time: 4 Hours Servings: 4
Ingredients:
- 1-pound chicken fillet, roughly cubed
- 1 teaspoon turmeric powder
- 1 teaspoon yellow curry paste

Directions:
- 1 oz Parmesan, grated
- ¼ cup butter

1. In the slow cooker, mix the chicken with the curry paste and the other ingredients and toss.
2. Close the lid and the chicken tenders for 4 hours on High. **Nutrition:** Calories 336, Fat 13.7, Fiber 2.6, Carbs 3.5, Protein 16.5

Paprika Almonds

Preparation Time: 10 Minutes
Cooking Time: 6 Hours Servings: 2 **Ingredients:**
- 1 cup almonds
- 1 tablespoon sweet paprika
- 1/3 cup water

Directions:
- ½ teaspoon Vanilla extract
- ¾ teaspoon ground ginger

1. In the slow cooker, mix the almonds with the other ingredients, toss and close the lid.
2. Cook the almonds for 6 hours on Low. Mix up the almonds every 1 hour.
Nutrition: Calories 126, Fat 4.3, Fiber 2.1, Carbs 9.1, Protein 5.2

Mixed Nuts

Preparation Time: 15 Minutes Cooking Time: 3 Hours Servings: 6
Ingredients:
- 1 cup almonds
- 1 cup walnuts
- 1 cup sunflower seeds
- 1/4 cup water

Directions:
- 2 tablespoons poppy seeds
- 1 teaspoon sweet paprika
- 1 teaspoon lemon zest, grated

1. In the slow cooker, mix the almonds with walnuts and the other ingredients, toss and close the lid.
2. Cook for 3 hours on High.
3. Divide into bowls and serve.
Nutrition: Calories 137, Fat 7.9, Fiber 2.3, Carbs 5.1, Protein 7.2

Beef and Zucchini Wraps

Preparation Time: 15 Minutes Cooking Time: 4 Hours Servings: 6
Ingredients:
- 6 keto tortillas
- 2 zucchinis, roughly cubed
- 1-pound beef sirloin, chopped
- 1 teaspoon sweet paprika

Directions:
- 5 tablespoons cream cheese
- 1 teaspoon butter
- 1 teaspoon garam masala

1. In the slow cooker, mix the zucchinis with the other ingredients except for the tortillas, stir and close the slow cooker lid.
2. Cook beef for 4 hours on High.
3. Divide this on each tortilla, wrap and serve.

Nutrition: Calories 278, Fat 8.3, Fiber 4.3, Carbs 8.8, Protein 23.7

Cauliflower Bites

Preparation Time: 10 Minutes **Cooking Time:** 3 Hours **Servings:** 5
Ingredients:
- 2 cups cauliflower florets
- ¾ cup coconut cream
- 4 oz Parmesan, grated

Directions:
- 1 teaspoon turmeric powder
- 1 teaspoon paprika
- 1 teaspoon butter, melted

1. In the slow cooker, mix the cauliflower with the cream and the other ingredients and close the lid.
2. Cook the cauliflower bites for 3 hours on High.

Nutrition: Calories 202, Fat 6.6, Fiber 5,.4, Carbs 2.9, Protein 9.2

Cheese Sticks

Preparation Time: 20 Minutes **Cooking Time:** 2 Hours and 30 Minutes **Servings:** 8
Ingredients:
- 4 eggs, beaten
- 1 cup Cheddar cheese, shredded
- 1 tablespoon fresh dill, chopped
- 1 tablespoon chives, chopped

Directions:
- 1 teaspoon turmeric powder
- 1 teaspoon butter, softened
- 1/3 cup almond flour
- 1 teaspoon salt

1. In the mixing bowl, mix up together beaten eggs, cheese, and the other ingredients. You should get a soft homogenous mixture.
2. Line the bottom of the slow cooker with the baking paper.
3. Transfer the cheese mixture to the slow cooker and flatten well.
4. Close the lid and bake it for 2.5 hours on High.
5. Then chill the cooked mixture very well and cut into the serving sticks.

Nutrition: Calories 304, Fat 8.3, Fiber 4.5, Carbs 1.6, Protein 7

Eggplant Bread

Preparation Time: 15 Minutes **Cooking Time:** 7 Hours **Servings:** 4
Ingredients:
- 2 eggplants, chopped
- 2 eggs, beaten
- 3 tablespoons coconut cream
- 1 teaspoon garam masala
- 2 tablespoons almond flour

Directions:
1. Line the slow cooker bottom with the baking paper.
- ½ teaspoon baking soda
- 1 teaspoon lime juice
- ½ teaspoon ground black pepper
- 1 teaspoon butter, melted

2. In the mixing bowl, mix up together eggs with the eggplants and the other ingredients, and stir really well.
3. Transfer the eggplant bread mixture to the slow cooker and flatten it well.
4. Close the lid and cook bread for 7 hours on Low.

Nutrition: Calories 186, Fat 12.1, Fiber 4.6, Carbs 11.2, Protein 7.5

Almond Granola

Preparation Time: 10 Minutes Cooking Time: 1 Hour and 30 Minutes Servings: 6
Ingredients:
- 1/3 cup coconut shred
- 1/4 cup almonds, chopped
- 2 eggs, whisked

Directions:
- 1 tablespoon almond flour
- 1 teaspoon Erythritol
- 1 teaspoon ground cinnamon

1. In the slow cooker, mix the almonds with the coconut and the other ingredients, stir and spread into the pot.
2. Cook granola on High for 1 hour.
3. Then mix up the granola mixture well and cook it for 30 minutes more.
4. Chill the cooked granola well and store it in the glass jar.

Nutrition: Calories 203, Fat 12.3, Fiber 3.1, Carbs 5.9, Protein 4.7

Chili Walnuts

Preparation Time: 10 Minutes Cooking Time: 2 Hours Servings: 3
Ingredients:
- 1 cup walnuts
- 1 teaspoon hot paprika
- 1 teaspoon salt

Directions:
- 1 egg white
- ½ teaspoon chili powder

1. Whisk the egg white, paprika, salt and chili until you get foam.
2. Coat walnuts in the egg white mixture.
3. Line the slow cooker bottom with baking paper and arrange coated walnuts.
4. Cook them for 2 hours on High.

Nutrition: Calories 270, Fat 10.1, Fiber 4.7, Carbs 6.3, Protein 5.8

Pork Bites

Preparation Time: 15 Minutes Cooking Time: 4 Hours Servings: 4
Ingredients:
- 1 cup pork stew meat, cubed
- 1 teaspoon keto tomato sauce
- 1 teaspoon chili flakes

Directions:
- ¼ cup heavy cream
- 1 teaspoon olive oil
- ½ teaspoon salt

1. In the slow cooker, mix the pork cubes with tomato paste and the other ingredients, close the lid and cook for 4 hours on High.
2. Divide into bowls and serve
Nutrition: Calories 283, Fat 20.2, Fiber 3.3, Carbs 1.4, Protein 14.5

Turkey Meatballs

Preparation Time: 15 Minutes Cooking Time: 4 Hours Servings: 3
Ingredients:
- ½ cup ground turkey meat
- 1 egg, whisked
- 1 teaspoon oregano, dried
- 1 teaspoon curry powder

Directions:
- ½ teaspoon ground black pepper
- ¼ teaspoon salt
- ¾ cup of coconut milk

1. In the mixing bowl, mix up together the meat with the egg and the other ingredients except for the coconut milk. Stir and shape small meatballs out of this mix.
2. Pour the coconut milk into the slow cooker, add the meatballs and toss gently.
3. Cook the meatballs for 4 hours on High.
Nutrition: Calories 273, Fat 16.7, Fiber 1.5, Carbs 4.1, Protein 11.8

Tomato Salmon Meatballs

Preparation Time: 15 Minutes Cooking Time: 3 Hours
Servings: 2
Ingredients:
- 6 oz salmon fillet, minced
- 1 tablespoon keto tomato sauce
- 1 teaspoon almond flour
- ½ teaspoon turmeric

Directions:
- ¾ teaspoon salt
- ¼ teaspoon sweet paprika
- ¼ cup organic almond milk
- 1 teaspoon butter

1. In a bowl, mix the salmon meat with the keto tomato sauce and the other ingredients except for the milk and butter, stir and make small meatballs.
2. Place them in the slow cooker, add butter and almond milk. Close the lid of the slow cooker.
3. Cook the appetizer for 3 hours on High
Nutrition: Calories 301, Fat 9.7, Fiber 2.7, Carbs 5.4, Protein 15.8

Pecans Bowl

Preparation Time: 7 Minutes Cooking Time: 60 Minutes Servings: 6
Ingredients:
- 6 pecans
- 1 teaspoon butter, melted

Directions:
- 1 tablespoon keto tomato sauce
- ½ teaspoon olive oil

1. In the slow cooker, mix the pecans with the keto tomato sauce and the other ingredients, toss and close the lid.
2. Cook pecans for 1 hour on High. Stir the pecans after 30 minutes of cooking and divide them into bowls at the end.

Nutrition: Calories 126, Fat 11.2, Fiber 1.5, Carbs 2, Protein 1.5

Sausage Dip

Preparation Time: 10 Minutes **Cooking Time:** 4 Hours **Servings:** 5
Ingredients:
- 1 cup Italian sausages, crumbled
- 1 tablespoon chives, chopped
- 1 teaspoon Italian seasoning
- 1 teaspoon sweet paprika

Directions:
- 1 cup Cheddar cheese, shredded
- 1 cup Mozzarella cheese, shredded
- ¼ cup heavy cream

1. In the slow cooker, mix the sausages with chives and the other ingredients and stir.
2. Close the lid and cook dip for 4 hours on Low.

Nutrition: Calories 304, Fat 24, Fiber 5.4, Carbs 6.5, Protein 13.8

Butter Pork Ribs

Preparation Time: 15 Minutes **Cooking Time:** 7 Hours **Servings:** 4
Ingredients:
- 10 oz pork ribs
- 3 tablespoons butter, soft
- 1/3 cup coconut cream

Directions:
- 1 teaspoon turmeric powder
- ½ teaspoon salt
- 1 teaspoon garlic powder

1. In the slow cooker, mix the pork with soft butter and the other ingredients.
2. Close the lid and cook the pork ribs for 7 hours on Low.

Nutrition: Calories 321, Fat 14.8, Fiber 4.5, Carbs 6.5, Protein 19.7

CHAPTER 6: FISH AND SEAFOOD

Mahi Mahi Taco Wraps

Preparation Time: 5 Minutes Cooking Time: 2 Hours
Servings: 6
Ingredients:
- 1-pound Mahi Mahi, wild-caught
- ½ cup cherry tomatoes
- 1 small green bell pepper, cored and sliced
- 1/4 of a medium red onion, thinly sliced
- ½ teaspoon garlic powder
- 1 teaspoon of sea salt
- ½ teaspoon ground black pepper
- 1 teaspoon chipotle pepper

Directions:
- ½ teaspoon dried oregano
- 1 teaspoon cumin
- 2 tablespoons avocado oil
- 1/4 cup chicken stock
- 1 medium avocado, diced
- 1 cup sour cream
- 6 large lettuce leaves

1. Grease a 6-quarts slow cooker with oil, place fish in it, and then pour in chicken stock.
2. Stir together garlic powder, salt, black pepper, chipotle pepper, oregano, and cumin, and then season fish with half of this mixture.
3. Layer fish with tomatoes, pepper, and onion, season with remaining spice mixture, and shut with lid.
4. Plug in the slow cooker and cook fish for 2 hours at high heat setting or until cooked through.
5. When done, evenly spoon fish among lettuce, top with avocado and sour cream, and serve.

Nutrition: Net Carbs: 2g; Calories: 193.6; Total Fat: 12g; Saturated Fat: 1.7g; Protein: 17g; Carbs: 5g; Fiber: 3g; Sugar: 2.5g

Shrimp Scampi

Preparation Time: 5 Minutes
Cooking Time: 2 Hours and 30 Minutes Servings: 4
Ingredients:
- 1 pound wild-caught shrimps, peeled & deveined
- 1 tablespoon minced garlic
- 1 teaspoon salt - ½ teaspoon ground black pepper
- 1/2 teaspoon red pepper flakes
- 2 tablespoons chopped parsley

Directions:
- 2 tablespoons avocado oil
- 2 tablespoons unsalted butter
- 1/2 cup white wine - 1 tablespoon lemon juice
- 1/4 cup chicken broth
- ½ cup grated parmesan cheese

1. Place all the ingredients except for shrimps and cheese in a 6-quart slow cooker and whisk until combined. Add shrimps and stir until evenly coated and shut with lid.
2. Plug in the slow cooker and cook for 1 hour and 30 minutes to 2 hours and 30 minutes at low heat setting or until cooked through. Then top with parmesan cheese and serve.

Nutrition: Net Carbs: 2g; Calories: 234; Total Fat: 14.7g; Saturated Fat: 2g; Protein: 23.3g; Carbs: 2.1g; Fiber: 0.1g; Sugar: 2g

Shrimp Tacos

Preparation Time: 5 Minutes Cooking Time: 3 Hours
Servings: 6
Ingredients:
- 1 pound medium wild-caught shrimp, peeled and tails off
- 12-ounce fire-roasted tomatoes, diced
- 1 small green bell pepper, chopped
- ½ cup chopped white onion
- 1 teaspoon minced garlic - ½ teaspoon of sea salt
- ½ teaspoon ground black pepper

Directions:
- ½ teaspoon red chili powder
- ½ teaspoon cumin
- ¼ teaspoon cayenne pepper
- 2 tablespoons avocado oil
- 1/2 cup salsa - 4 tablespoons chopped cilantro
- 1 ½ cup sour cream
- 2 mediums avocado, diced

1. Rinse shrimps, layer into a 6-quarts slow cooker, and drizzle with oil. Add tomatoes, stir until mixed, then add peppers and remaining ingredients except for sour cream and avocado and stir until combined. Plug in the slow cooker, shut with lid, and cook for 2 to 3 hours at low heat setting or 1 hour and 30 minutes to 2 hours at high heat setting or until shrimps turn pink.
2. When done, serve shrimps with avocado and sour cream.

Nutrition: Net Carbs: 4.2g; Calories: 369; Total Fat: 27.5g; Saturated Fat: 7.9g; Protein: 21.2g; Carbs: 9.2g; Fiber: 5g; Sugar: 5g

Fish Curry

Preparation Time: 5 Minutes
Cooking Time: 4 Hours and 30 Minutes Servings: 6
Ingredients:
- 2.2 pounds wild-caught white fish fillet, cubed - 18-ounce spinach leaves
- 4 tablespoons red curry paste, organic

Directions:
- 14-ounce coconut cream, unsweetened and full-fat - 14-ounce water

1. Plug in a 6-quart slow cooker and let preheat at high heat setting. In the meantime, whisk together coconut cream and water until smooth. Place fish into the slow cooker, spread with curry paste, and then pour in coconut cream mixture.
2. Shut with lid, then cook for 2 hours at high heat setting or 4 hours using the low heat setting until tender. Then add spinach and continue cooking for 20 to 30 minutes or until spinach leaves wilt.
3. Serve straight away.

Nutrition: Net Carbs: 4.8g; Calories: 323; Total Fat: 51.5g; Saturated Fat: 23.3g; Protein: 41.3g; Carbs: 7g; Fiber: 2.2g; Sugar: 2.3g

Salmon with Creamy Lemon Sauce

Preparation Time: 5 Minutes - Cooking Time: 2 Hours and 15 Minutes Servings: 6
Ingredients:
For the Salmon:
- 2 pounds wild-caught salmon fillet, skin- on - 1 teaspoon garlic powder
- 1 ½ teaspoon salt - 1 teaspoon ground black pepper - 1/2 teaspoon red chili powder - 1 teaspoon Italian Seasoning
- 1 lemon, sliced

Directions:

- 1 lemon, juiced
- 2 tablespoons avocado oil - 1 cup chicken broth

For the Creamy Lemon Sauce:
- Chopped parsley, for garnish
- 1/8 teaspoon lemon zest - 1/4 cup heavy cream - 1/4 cup grated parmesan cheese

1. Line a 6-quart slow cooker with parchment sheet spread its bottom with lemon slices, top with salmon and drizzle with oil. Stir together garlic powder, salt, black pepper, red chili powder, Italian seasoning, and oil until combined and rub this mixture all over salmon. Pour lemon juice and broth around the fish and shut with lid. Plug in the slow cooker and cook for 2 hours at a low heat setting.
2. In the meantime, set the oven at 400 degrees F and let preheat.
3. When fish is done, lift out an inner pot of slow cooker, place into the oven and cook for 5 to 8 minutes or until the top is nicely browned. Lift out fish using a parchment sheet and keep it warm.
4. Transfer juices from slow cooker to a medium skillet pan, place it over medium-high heat, then bring to boil and cook for 1 minute. Turn heat to a low level, whisk the cream into the sauce along with lemon zest and parmesan cheese and cook for 2 to 3 minutes or until thickened.
5. Cut salmon in pieces, then top each piece with lemon sauce and serve.

Nutrition: Net Carbs: 6g; Calories: 340; Total Fat: 20g; Saturated Fat: 4g; Protein: 32g; Carbs: 8g; Fiber: 2g; Sugar: 2g

Salmon with Lemon-Caper Sauce

Preparation Time: 5 Minutes Cooking Time: 1 Hour and 30 Minutes
Servings: 4
Ingredients:
- 1 pound wild-caught salmon fillet
- 2 teaspoon capers, rinsed and mashed
- 1 teaspoon minced garlic
- 1 teaspoon salt
- ½ teaspoon ground black pepper

Directions:
- 1/2 teaspoon dried oregano
- 1 teaspoon lemon zest
- 2 tablespoons lemon juice
- 4 tablespoons unsalted butter

1. Cut salmon into four pieces, then season with salt and black pepper and sprinkle lemon zest on top.
2. Line a 6-quart slow cooker with parchment paper, place seasoned salmon pieces on it, and shut with lid.
3. Plug in the slow cooker and cook for 1 hour and 30 minutes or until salmon is cooked through.
4. When 10 minutes of cooking time is left, prepare lemon-caper sauce and for this, place a small saucepan over low heat, add butter and let it melt.
5. Then add capers, garlic, lemon juice, stir until mixed, and simmer for 1 minute.
6. Remove saucepan from heat and stir in oregano.
7. When salmon is cooked, spoon lemon-caper sauce on it and serve.

Nutrition: Net Carbs: 2.4g; Calories: 368.5; Total Fat: 26.6g; Saturated Fat: 10.1g; Protein: 19.5g; Carbs: 2.7g; Fiber: 0.3g; Sugar: 2g

Spicy Barbecue Shrimp

Preparation Time: 5 Minutes Cooking Time: 1 Hour and 30 Minutes
Servings: 6
Ingredients:
- 1 1/2 pounds large wild-caught shrimp, unpeeled
- 1 green onion, chopped
- 1 teaspoon minced garlic
- 1 ½ teaspoon salt
- ¾ teaspoon ground black pepper

Directions:
- 1 teaspoon Cajun seasoning
- 1 tablespoon hot pepper sauce
- ¼ cup Worcestershire Sauce
- 1 lemon, juiced
- 2 tablespoons avocado oil
- 1/2 cup unsalted butter, chopped

1. Place all the ingredients except for shrimps in a 6-quart slow cooker and whisk until mixed.
2. Plug in the slow cooker then shut with lid and cook for 30 minutes at a high heat setting.
3. Then take out ½ cup of this sauce and reserve.
4. Add shrimps to slow cooker.

Nutrition: Net Carbs: 2.4g; Calories: 321; Total Fat: 21.4g; Saturated Fat: 10.6g; Protein: 27.3g; Carbs: 4.8g; Fiber: 2.4g; Sugar: 1.2g

Lemon Dill Halibut

Preparation Time: 5 Minutes **Cooking Time:** 2 Hours
Servings: 2
Ingredients:
- 12-ounce wild-caught halibut fillet
- 1 teaspoon salt
- ½ teaspoon ground black pepper

Directions:
- 1 1/2 teaspoon dried dill
- 1 tablespoon fresh lemon juice
- 3 tablespoons avocado oil

1. Cut an 18-inch piece of aluminum foil, halibut fillet in the middle and then season with salt and black pepper.
2. Whisk together remaining ingredients, drizzle this mixture over halibut, then crimp the foil's edges and place it into a 6-quart slow cooker.
3. Plug in the slow cooker, shut with lid, and cook for 1 hour and 30 minutes or 2 hours at high heat setting or until cooked through.
4. When done, carefully open the crimped edges and check the fish. It should be tender and flaky.
5. Serve straight away.

Nutrition: Net Carbs: 0g; Calories: 321.5; Total Fat: 21.4g; Saturated Fat: 7.2g; Protein: 32.1g; Carbs: 0g; Fiber: 0g; Sugar: 0.6g

Coconut Cilantro Curry Shrimp

Preparation Time: 5 Minutes
Cooking Time: 2 Hours and 30 Minutes Servings: 4
Ingredients:
- 1 pound wild-caught shrimp, peeled and deveined
- 2 ½ teaspoon lemon garlic seasoning
- 2 tablespoons red curry paste

Directions:
- 4 tablespoons chopped cilantro
- 30 ounces coconut milk, unsweetened
- 16 ounces of water

1. Whisk together all the ingredients except for shrimps and two tablespoons cilantro and add to a 4-quart slow cooker.
2. Plug in the slow cooker, shut with lid, and cook for 2 hours at high heat setting or 4 hours at low heat setting.
3. Then add shrimps, toss until evenly coated and cook for 20 to 30 minutes at high heat settings or until shrimps are pink.
4. Garnish shrimps with remaining cilantro and serve.

Nutrition: Net Carbs: 1.9g; Calories: 160.7; Total Fat: 8.2g; Saturated Fat: 8.1g; Protein: 19.3g; Carbs: 2.4g; Fiber: 0.5g; Sugar: 1.4g

Shrimp in Marinara Sauce

Preparation Time: 5 Minutes
Cooking Time: 5 Hours and 10 Minutes Servings: 5
Ingredients:
- 1 pound cooked wild-caught shrimps, peeled and deveined
- 14.5-ounce crushed tomatoes
- ½ teaspoon minced garlic
- 1 teaspoon salt
- 1/2 teaspoon seasoned salt
- ¼ teaspoon ground black pepper

Directions:
- ½ teaspoon crushed red pepper flakes
- 1/2 teaspoon dried basil
- 1/2 teaspoon dried oregano
- ½ tablespoons avocado oil
- 6-ounce chicken broth
- 2 tablespoon minced parsley
- 1/2 cup grated Parmesan cheese

1. Place all the ingredients except for shrimps, parsley, and cheese in a 4-quart slow cooker and stir well. Then plug in the slow cooker, shut with lid, and cook for 4 to 5 hours at low heat setting.
2. Then add shrimps and parsley, stir until mixed and cook for 10 minutes at high heat setting.
3. Garnish shrimps with cheese and serve.

Nutrition: Net Carbs: 5.7g; Calories: 358.8; Total Fat: 25.1g; Saturated Fat: 4.3g; Protein: 26g; Carbs: 7.2g; Fiber: 1.5g; Sugar: 3.6g

Garlic Shrimp

Preparation Time: 5 Minutes Cooking Time: 60 Minutes
Servings: 5
Ingredients:
For the Garlic Shrimp:
- 1 1/2 pounds large wild-caught shrimp, peeled and deveined
- 1/4 teaspoon ground black pepper
- 1/8 teaspoon ground cayenne pepper
- 2 ½ teaspoons minced garlic
- 1/4 cup avocado oil
- 4 tablespoons unsalted butter For the Seasoning:

Directions:
- 1 teaspoon onion powder
- 1 tablespoon garlic powder
- 1 tablespoon salt
- 2 teaspoons ground black pepper
- 1 tablespoon paprika
- 1 teaspoon cayenne pepper
- 1 teaspoon dried oregano
- 1 teaspoon dried thyme

1. Stir together all the ingredients for seasoning, garlic, oil, and butter and add to a 4-quart slow cooker.
2. Plug in the slow cooker, shut with lid, and cook for 25 to 30 minutes at high heat setting or until cooked. Then add shrimps, toss until evenly coated, and continue cooking for 20 to 30 minutes at high heat setting or until shrimps are pink.

3. When done, transfer shrimps to a serving plate, top with sauce, and serve.
Nutrition: Net Carbs: 1.2g; Calories: 233.6; Total Fat: 11.7g; Saturated Fat: 1.3g; Protein: 30.9g; Carbs: 1.2g; Fiber: 0g; Sugar: 0g

Poached Salmon

Preparation Time: 5 Minutes
Cooking Time: 3 Hours and 35 Minutes Servings: 4
Ingredients:
- 4 steaks of wild-caught salmon
- 1 medium white onion, peeled and sliced
- 2 teaspoons minced garlic
- 1/2 teaspoon salt
- 1/8 teaspoon ground white pepper

Directions:
- 1/2 teaspoon dried dill weed
- 2 tablespoons avocado oil
- 2 tablespoons unsalted butter
- 2 tablespoons lemon juice
- 1 cup of water

1. Place butter in a 4-quart slow cooker, then adds salmon and drizzle with oil.
2. Place remaining ingredients in a medium saucepan, stir until mixed and bring the mixture to boil over high heat.
3. Then pour this mixture all over salmon and shut with lid.
4. Plug in the slow cooker and cook salmon for 3 hours and 30 minutes at low heat setting or until salmon is tender.
5. Serve straight away.

Nutrition: Net Carbs: 2.8g; Calories: 310; Total Fat: 20g; Saturated Fat: 4.8g; Protein: 30.2g; Carbs: 3.1g; Fiber: 0.3g; Sugar: 1.2g

Lemon Pepper Tilapia

Preparation Time: 5 Minutes Cooking Time: 3 Hours
Servings: 6
Ingredients:
- 6 wild-caught Tilapia fillets
- 4 teaspoons lemon-pepper seasoning, divided

Directions:
- 6 tablespoons unsalted butter, divided
- 1/2 cup lemon juice, fresh

1. Cut a large piece of aluminum foil for each fillet and then arrange them on clean working space.
2. Place each fillet in the middle of the foil, then season with lemon-pepper seasoning, drizzle with lemon juice, and top with one tablespoon butter.
3. Gently crimp the edges of foil to form a packet and place it into a 6-quart slow cooker.
4. Plug in the slow cooker, shut with lid, and cook for 3 hours at high heat setting or until cooked through.
5. When done, carefully remove packets from the slow cooker and open the crimped edges and check the fish. It should be tender and flaky.
6. Serve straight away.

Nutrition: Net Carbs: 1.2 g; Calories: 201.2; Total Fat: 12.9g; Saturated Fat: 9.1g; Protein: 19.6g; Carbs: 1.5g; Fiber: 0.3g; Sugar: 0.7g

Clam Chowder

Preparation Time: 5 Minutes Cooking Time: 6 Hours
Servings: 6

Ingredients:
- 20-ounce wild-caught baby clams, with juice
- ½ cup chopped scallion
- ½ cup chopped celery
- 1 teaspoon salt

Directions:
- 1 teaspoon ground black pepper
- 1 teaspoon dried thyme
- 1 tablespoon avocado oil
- 2 cups coconut cream, full-fat
- 2 cups chicken broth

1. Grease a 6-quart slow cooker with oil, then add ingredients and stir until mixed.
2. Plug in the slow cooker, shut with lid, and cook for 4 to 6 hours at low heat setting or until cooked through.
3. Serve straight away.

Nutrition: Net Carbs: 6.8g; Calories: 357; Total Fat: 28.9g; Saturated Fat: 13.2g; Protein: 15.2g; Carbs: 8.9g; Fiber: 2.1g; Sugar: 3.9g

Soy-Ginger Steamed Pompano

Preparation Time: 5 Minutes Cooking Time: 60 Minutes
Servings: 4

Ingredients:
- 1 wild-caught whole pompano, gutted and scaled
- 1 bunch scallion, diced
- 1 bunch cilantro, chopped
- 3 teaspoons minced garlic

Directions:
- 1 tablespoon grated ginger
- 1 tablespoon swerve sweetener
- ¼ cup of soy sauce
- ¼ cup white wine
- ¼ cup sesame oil

1. Place scallions in a 6-quart slow cooker and top with fish.
2. Whisk together the remaining ingredients, except for cilantro, and pour the mixture all over the fish.
3. Plug in the slow cooker, shut with lid, and cook for 1 hour at high heat setting or until cooked through.
4. Garnish with cilantro and serve.

Nutrition: Net Carbs: 3.5g; Calories: 202.5; Total Fat: 24.2g; Saturated Fat: 6g; Protein: 22.7g; Carbs: 4g; Fiber: 0.5g; Sugar: 1.1g

CHAPTER 7: POULTRY

Chicken Noodle Soup

Preparation Time: 15 Minutes Cooking Time: 4 Hours Servings: 6
Ingredients:
- 8 cups chicken broth
- 1 lb. chicken breast fillet
- 1 onion, diced
- 2 cloves garlic, minced
- 3 stalks celery, chopped
- 3 carrots, sliced
- 1 tablespoon rosemary
- 1 tablespoon thyme
- 1 teaspoon salt
- 8 oz. egg noodles

Directions:
1. First, pour the chicken broth into your slow cooker.
2. Add the chicken breast fillet, onion, garlic, celery, and carrots.
3. Season with the rosemary, thyme, and salt.
4. Cover the pot.
5. Next, cook on low for 8 hours or on high for 4 hours.
6. In the last 15 minutes of cooking, take out the chicken breast, and shred it using a fork.
7. Then, put the shredded chicken back in the pot.
8. Add the egg noodles.
9. Continue cooking.
10. Serve in soup bowls.

Nutrition: Calories 273, Fat 8.4 g, Saturated Fat 2.3 g, Carbohydrate 16.7 g, Dietary Fiber 2.2 g, Protein 30.7 g, Cholesterol 78 mg, Sugars 3.5 g, Sodium 1501 mg, Potassium 633 mg

Chicken Enchilada Casserole

Preparation Time: 5 Minutes Cooking Time: 4 or 8 Hours
Servings: 6
Ingredients:
- 1 lb. chicken breast fillet, diced
- Salt and pepper to taste
- 1 onion, diced
- 1 red bell pepper, diced
- 1 green bell pepper, diced
- 15 oz. canned black beans, drained
- 15 oz. sweet corn kernels, drained
- 20 oz. canned enchilada sauce
- 1 cup taco cheese, shredded
- 10 tortillas, sliced into strips

Directions:
1. First, season the diced chicken with salt and pepper.
2. Add these to the slow cooker. Stir in the onion, bell peppers, black beans, corn kernels, and enchilada sauce.
3. Next, mix well. Cover the pot. Then, cook on high for 4 hours or on low for 8 hours.
4. Top the dish with the tortilla strips and cheese.

Nutrition: Calories 493, Fat 7.9 g, Saturated Fat 2 g, Carbohydrate 66.8 g, Dietary Fiber 14.2 g, Protein 40.1 g, Cholesterol 67 mg, Sugars 4.6 g, Sodium 88 mg, Potassium 1411 mg

Chicken Basque

Preparation Time: 5 Minutes
Cooking Time: 4 Hours and 30 Minutes Servings: 4
Ingredients:
- 4 chicken breast fillets - Salt and pepper to taste - 1 tablespoon olive oil
- 1 cup Spanish chorizo, sliced into rounds
- 12 oz. beer
- 2 tablespoons red wine vinegar
- 1 ½ cups reduced-sodium chicken broth

Directions:
- 1 onion, sliced into wedges
- 8 cloves garlic, peeled
- 1 red bell pepper, chopped
- ½ teaspoon cumin - 1 teaspoon smoked paprika - 2 bay leaves
- 4 cups baby spinach

1. First, sprinkle the chicken with salt and pepper. Pour the olive oil into a pan over medium high heat.
2. Add the chicken to the pan. Next, cook for 3 to 4 minutes per side.
3. Stir in the chorizo slices. Cook for 2 minutes.
4. Transfer the chicken and chorizo to your slow cooker.
5. Pour in the beer. Next, scrape the bottom of the pan.
6. Add the vinegar, chicken broth, onion, garlic, red bell pepper, cumin paprika, and bay leaves to the pot. Seal the pot.
7. Then, cook on low for 4 hours.
8. Stir in the spinach.
9. Discard the bay leaves before serving.

Nutrition: Calories 420, Fat 22.1 g, Saturated Fat 3.8 g, Carbohydrate 28 g, Dietary Fiber 3 g, Protein 21.8 g, Cholesterol 48 mg, Sugars 6.2 g, Sodium 1032 mg, Potassium 721 mg

Chicken Curry

Preparation Time: 5 Minutes
Cooking Time: 6 Hours and 30 Minutes Servings: 4
Ingredients:
- Chicken - 16 oz. chicken breast fillet, sliced into cubes
- 1 tablespoon garlic, minced
- ½ teaspoon garlic powder
- 3 tablespoons green curry paste
- 2 tablespoons Thai basil
- ½ teaspoon chili powder
- 2 tablespoons lime juice

Directions:
- Salt and pepper to taste
- Onion and peppers
- 1 red onion, sliced
- 1 red bell pepper, sliced
- 1 green bell pepper, sliced
- 2 tablespoons coconut oil
- Salt and pepper to taste
- Brown rice - 4 cups cooked brown rice

1. First, add the chicken breast cubes to your slow cooker. Sprinkle the minced garlic on top. Cover the pot. Next, cook on high for 2 hours or low for 6 hours.
2. Uncover the pot carefully. Stir in the rest of the ingredients for the chicken curry.
3. Simmer for 30 minutes. In a pan over medium heat, add the coconut oil.

4. Next, cook the onion and bell peppers for 2 to 3 minutes, stirring often.
5. Season with salt and pepper. Then, add them to the chicken curry. Serve with the cooked brown rice.

Nutrition: Calories 440, Fat 6 g, Saturated fat 0 g, Carbohydrates 33 g, Fiber 4 g, Protein 30 g, Cholesterol 0 mg, Sugars 1 g, Sodium 220 mg, Potassium 135 mg

Chicken & Pumpkin Chili

Preparation Time: 5 Minutes Cooking Time: 4 Hours or 8 Hours
Servings: 6
Ingredients:
- ½ cup onion, chopped
- 1 tablespoon garlic, minced
- 1 cup red bell pepper, chopped
- ½ cup celery, chopped
- ½ cup carrot, chopped
- 1 ½ lb. chicken thigh fillet, sliced into cubes

Directions:
- 15 oz. chickpeas, rinsed and drained
- 15 oz. canned pumpkin puree
- 14 oz. roasted diced tomatoes
- 14 oz. low-sodium chicken broth
- 1 ½ teaspoons dried oregano, crushed
- 4 teaspoons chili powder
- Salt and pepper to taste - Hot sauce

1. First, add all the ingredients except the hot sauce to your slow cooker. Seal the pot. Then, cook on high for 4 hours or low for 8 hours.
2. Drizzle with the hot sauce before serving.

Nutrition: Calories 526, Fat 13.3 g, Saturated Fat 2.9 g, Carbohydrate 54.2 g, Dietary Fiber 16 g, Protein 48.6 g, Cholesterol 101 mg, Sugars 12 g, Sodium 169 mg, Potassium 1190 mg

Maple Chicken & Veggies

Preparation Time: 5 Minutes
Cooking Time: 5 Hours and 30 Minutes Servings: 4
Ingredients:
- 1 tablespoon maple syrup
- 3 tablespoons balsamic vinegar
- ½ cup low-sodium chicken broth
- 5 teaspoon tapioca (quick-cooking), crushed
- Salt and pepper to taste

Directions:
- 1 lb. potatoes, sliced in half
- 4 carrots, sliced
- 3 stalks celery, sliced
- 1 onion, sliced into wedges
- 8 chicken drumsticks, skin removed
- 2 teaspoons fresh rosemary, snipped

1. First, add the maple syrup, balsamic vinegar, chicken broth, tapioca, salt and pepper to your slow cooker. Nestle the chicken on top.
2. Cover the pot. Next, cook on low for 10 hours or on high for 5 hours.
3. Transfer the chicken mixture to a serving plate.
4. Garnish with the rosemary and serve.

Nutrition: Calories 380, Fat 11 g, Saturated fat 3.5 g, Carbohydrates 20 g, Fiber 10 g, Protein 33 g, Cholesterol 102 mg, Sugars 8 g, Sodium 700 mg, Potassium 452 mg

Chicken Parmesan Soup

Preparation Time: 20 Minutes Cooking Time: 4 Hours Servings: 4
Ingredients:
- ½ white onion, chopped
- 4 cloves garlic, minced
- 1 green bell pepper, chopped
- 14 oz. canned crushed tomatoes
- ½ lb. chicken breast fillet
- 5 cups reduced-sodium chicken broth
- 2 teaspoons fresh oregano, chopped

Directions:
- 2 tablespoons fresh basil, chopped
- ½ cup Parmesan cheese, shredded
- ¼ teaspoon red pepper flakes
- Salt and pepper to taste
- 4 oz. penne pasta
- Chopped parsley for garnish

1. Add the onion, garlic, bell pepper, crushed tomatoes, chicken breast fillet, chicken broth, oregano, basil, Parmesan cheese, red pepper flakes, salt, and pepper.
2. Seal the pot. Next, cook on high for 3 hours or low for 7 hours.
3. Take the chicken out of the slow cooker.
4. Place it on a cutting board. Shred using a fork.
5. Next, put it back in the slow cooker. Add the pasta to the pot.
6. Cook on high for 30 minutes. Lastly, garnish with chopped parsley.

Nutrition: Calories 312, Fat 13 g, Saturated fat 7 g, Carbohydrates 20 g, Fiber 2 g, Protein 31 g, Cholesterol 71 mg, Sugars 4 g, Sodium 890 mg, Potassium 601 mg

Sweet Spicy Chicken

Preparation Time: 20 Minutes Cooking Time: 2 Hours Servings: 6
Ingredients:
- ½ cup honey
- ½ cup coconut aminos
- ½ cup hot pepper sauce
- 2 tablespoons garlic, minced

Directions:
- 1 ½ lb. chicken breast fillet, sliced into cubes
- 1 ½ tablespoons cornstarch

1. First, in a bowl, combine the garlic, coconut aminos, hot pepper sauce, and honey.
2. Add the chicken breast fillet to your slow cooker.
3. Pour the sauce over the chicken.
4. Cover the pot. Next, cook on high for 2 hours or on low for 6 hours.
5. Stir in the cornstarch. Then, mix until fully combined.
6. Simmer until sauce has thickened.

Nutrition: Calories 321, Fat 8.4 g, Saturated Fat 2.3 g, Carbohydrate 27.7 g, Dietary Fiber 0.1 g, Protein 33.1 g, Cholesterol 101 mg, Sugars 23.2 g, Sodium 109 mg, Potassium 302 mg

Chicken Cordon Bleu Soup

Preparation Time: 5 Minutes
Cooking Time: 3 Hours and 40 Minutes Servings: 8
Ingredients:
- 6 cups reduced-sodium chicken broth
- 2 cloves garlic, minced

- 2 chicken breast fillets, diced
- ½ white onion, chopped
- ½ cup carrots, shredded
- 1 cup ham, diced

Directions:
1. First, pour the broth into your slow cooker.
- 1 teaspoon dried tarragon
- Salt and pepper to taste
- 1 cup low-fat milk
- ½ cup low-fat Swiss cheese, grated
- 2 tablespoons butter, melted
- 2 tablespoons flour

2. Stir in the onion, garlic, carrots, chicken breast, ham, dried tarragon, salt and pepper.
3. Seal the pot.
4. Next, cook on low for 5 hours or on high for 3 hours.
5. In a pan over medium heat, add the milk and stir in the cheese.
6. Cook while stirring until cheese has melted.
7. In a bowl, mix the flour and butter.
8. Next, add the cheese mixture and flour mixture to the pot.
9. Mix well. Simmer for 10 minutes.

Nutrition: Calories 211, Fat 12 g, Saturated fat 5 g, Carbohydrates 8 g, Fiber 1 g, Protein 19 g, Cholesterol 53 mg, Sugars 3 g, Sodium 546 mg, Potassium 450 mg

Honey Garlic Chicken

Preparation Time: 15 Minutes Cooking Time: 4 Hours Servings: 8
Ingredients:
- 4 chicken breast fillets
- ¼ cup olive oil
- 2 tablespoons garlic, minced

Directions:
- Salt and pepper to taste
- ½ cup reduced-sodium soy sauce
- 1/3 cup honey

1. First, add the chicken to your slow cooker. Coat evenly with the olive oil. Sprinkle the garlic on top.
2. Next, season with salt and pepper. Pour in the soy sauce and honey.
3. Seal the pot.
4. Then, cook on high for 4 hours or low for 8 hours.
5. Slice before serving.

Nutrition: Calories 257, Fat 10 g, Saturated fat 2 g, Carbohydrates 13 g, Fiber 0 g, Protein 28 g, Cholesterol 86 mg, Sugars 12 g, Sodium 788 mg, Potassium 413 mg

Chicken & Corn Chowder

Preparation Time: 5 Minutes
Cooking Time: 3 Hours and 30 Minutes Servings: 8
Ingredients:
- 1 tablespoon olive oil
- 1 ½ lb. chicken breast fillet
- Salt and pepper to taste
- 1 cup onion, diced - 1 cup corn kernels
- 1 potato, sliced into cubes
- ½ cup celery, diced - ½ cup carrots, diced

Directions:

1. First, in a pan, heat the olive oil over medium heat.
2. Season the chicken with salt and pepper.
- ½ cup heavy cream
- 1 ½ cups low-sodium chicken broth
- 14 oz. cream-style corn
- 1 ½ teaspoons dried thyme
- 6 slices bacon, cooked crisp and chopped
- Chopped parsley for garnish
3. Next, gradually cook the chicken until browned on both sides.
4. Add the chicken and the rest of the ingredients except parsley and bacon to the slow cooker.
5. Cover the pot. Next, cook on high for 3 hours or low for 6 hours.
6. Transfer the chicken to a cutting board.
7. Slice the chicken. Set aside. Pour the mixture into a blender.
8. Pulse until smooth. Then, put the mixture into a pan.
9. Reheat for a few minutes.
10. Serve in bowls.
11. Top with the crispy bacon bits, chicken slices, and parsley.

Nutrition: Calories 248.9, Fat 8.1 g, Saturated Fat 4.1 g, Carbohydrates 21.3 g, Fiber 2.2 g, Protein 24 g, Cholesterol 73.6 mg, Sugar 4.4 g, Sodium 603.6 mg, Potassium 780 mg

Moroccan Chicken

Preparation Time: 15 Minutes Cooking Time: 9 Hours Servings: 6
Ingredients:
Sweet Potatoes
- 2 sweet potatoes, sliced into cubes
- ½ tablespoon olive oil
- ½ tablespoon chili powder
- 1 teaspoon garlic powder Chicken
- 1 teaspoon ground ginger
- 1 teaspoon turmeric
- 1 tablespoon cumin
- ½ tablespoon chili powder
- 1 ½ teaspoons garlic powder
- Salt to taste
- 6 chicken thighs
- 3 tablespoons olive oil, divided

Directions:
1. Preheat your oven to 400 degrees F.
2. Spread the sweet potatoes in a baking pan.
3. Coat the sweet potato with the olive oil.
4. Season with the chili powder and garlic powder.
- 1 white onion, chopped
- ½ cup green olives, chopped
- ¼ cup raisins
- ½ cup chicken broth Couscous
- 1 cup of water
- 1 cup couscous, uncooked
- 2 tablespoons lemon juice
- 1 teaspoon lemon zest
- ¼ cup fresh cilantro, chopped
- ¼ cup parsley, chopped Toppings
- Feta cheese, crumbled

5. Bake the sweet potatoes in the oven for 20 minutes.
6. In a bowl, mix the ground ginger, turmeric, cumin, chili powder, garlic powder, and salt.
7. Season the chicken with this spice mixture.
8. Brown the chicken in 2 tablespoons olive oil on a pan over medium heat.
9. Stir in the rest of the chicken ingredients in the pan.
10. Cook for 2 minutes, stirring often.
11. Transfer the mixture to the slow cooker.
12. Seal the pot.
13. Cook on low for 8 hours.
14. While waiting, add the water to a pot over medium high heat.
15. Bring to a boil.
16. Turn off the heat.
17. Add the couscous to the hot water.
18. Let it sit for 5 minutes.
19. Fluff the couscous using a fork. Set aside.
20. Serve the chicken with the baked sweet potatoes and couscous.
21. Top with the feta cheese.

Nutrition: Calories 314, Fat 11.8 g, Saturated Fat 2 g, Carbohydrate 44.8 g, Dietary Fiber 4.7 g, Protein 8.4 g, Cholesterol 10 mg, Sugars 5 g, Sodium 121 mg, Potassium 642 mg

Quinoa Chicken Primavera

Preparation Time: 5 Minutes
Cooking Time: 4 Hours and 30 Minutes Servings: 8
Ingredients:
- 7 cups chicken broth, divided
- 1 lb. chicken breast fillets, sliced into cubes
- 1 ½ cups quinoa, rinsed and drained
- 4 cloves garlic
- ½ teaspoon dried parsley
- Salt and pepper to taste

Directions:
For serving
- 2 ½ cups peas
- 6 oz. pesto
- 1 teaspoon lemon juice
- 1 cup asparagus, sliced and steamed
- Fresh parsley, chopped
- Parmesan cheese, shaved

1. First, pour 4 cups chicken broth into your slow cooker. Add the chicken breast, quinoa, garlic, dried parsley, salt, and pepper.
2. Seal the pot. Cook on low for 4 hours. Next, stir in the remaining broth along with the peas, pesto, and lemon juice. Cook for 10 minutes. Stir in the asparagus before serving.
3. Lastly, top with the parsley and Parmesan cheese.

Nutrition: Calories 355, Fat 14.7 g, Saturated fat 2 g, Carbohydrates 31.8 g, Fiber 5.4 g, Protein 24.1 g, Cholesterol 45.7 mg, Sugars 5.4 g, Sodium 884 mg, Potassium 570 mg

Chicken with Mint Garlic Sauce & Lentils

Preparation Time: 5 Minutes
Cooking Time: 3 Hours and 40 Minutes Servings: 6
Ingredients:
- 3 tablespoons olive oil - 3 mint leaves
- ½ cup basil leaves - ¼ cup sweet onion, chopped - 3 cloves garlic, peeled
- ¼ cup of orange juice - ½ teaspoon smoked paprika - ½ teaspoon chili pepper

Directions:
- Salt and pepper to taste - 1 ½ cups vegetable broth - 1 tablespoon butter
- 1 cup green lentils
- 1 ½ lb. chicken breast fillet
- ½ avocado, mashed - ¼ cup sour cream

1. First, add the olive oil, mint leaves, basil leaves, sweet onion, garlic, orange juice, paprika, chili pepper, salt, and pepper to your food processor. Pulse until smooth. Pour the broth into your slow cooker.
2. Stir in the butter and lentils. Next, add the chicken on top.
3. Spread the mint mixture on top of the chicken. Cover the pot.
4. Cook on high for 3 hours or on low for 6 hours. Then, in a bowl, mix the mashed avocado and sour cream. Serve the chicken, lentils, and sauce on a platter. Top with the avocado cream.

Nutrition: Calories 406, Fat 14.8 g, Saturated fat 3.5 g, Carbohydrates 27.9 g, Fiber 4.4 g, Protein 40.5 g, Cholesterol 105 mg, Sugars 2.8 g, Sodium 462 mg, Potassium 556 mg

Orange Chicken

Preparation Time: 5 Minutes
Cooking Time: 2 Hours and 40 Minutes Servings: 4
Ingredients:
- 1 cup reduced-sodium chicken broth
- ½ cup of orange juice
- 2 cloves garlic, minced
- ¼ cup honey
- ¼ cup brown sugar
- ½ cup of soy sauce
- ½ cup of rice vinegar
- 1 teaspoon red pepper flakes

Directions:
- ¼ teaspoon ground ginger
- 2 tablespoons orange zest
- Pepper to taste
- 2 lb. chicken breast fillet
- ¼ cup cornstarch
- Cilantro, chopped
- Green onion, chopped
- Sesame seeds

1. First, add the chicken broth, orange juice, garlic, honey, brown sugar, soy sauce, rice vinegar, red pepper flakes, ground ginger, orange zest, and pepper to a bowl.
2. Mix well. Pour half of the mixture into your slow cooker.
3. Add the chicken breast fillet to the pot. Pour the rest of the mixture on top of the chicken.
4. Lock the lid in place. Next, cook on high for 2 hours or low for 4 hours.
5. Stir in the cornstarch to the mixture. Cook on high for 30 minutes.
6. Slice the chicken into smaller pieces and then return to the pot.
7. Lastly, top with the cilantro, green onion, and sesame seeds before serving.

Nutrition: Calories 451, Fat 6 g, Saturated fat 1 g, Carbohydrates 44 g, Fiber 2 g, Protein 51 g, Cholesterol 145 mg, Sugars 33 g, Sodium 850 mg, Potassium 1048 mg

Aromatic Jalapeno Wings

Preparation Time: 10 Minutes Cooking Time: 3 Hours Servings: 4
Ingredients:
- 1 jalapeño pepper, diced
- ½ cup of fresh cilantro, diced
- 3 tablespoon of coconut oil

- Juice from 1 lime
- 2 garlic cloves, peeled and minced

Directions:
- Salt and black pepper ground, to taste
- 2 lbs. chicken wings
- Lime wedges, to serve
- Mayonnaise, to serve

1. Start by throwing all the Ingredients: into the large bowl and mix well.
2. Cover the wings and marinate them in the refrigerator for 2 hours.
3. Now add the wings along with their marinade into the Slow cooker.
4. Cover it and cook for 3 hours on Low Settings. Garnish as desired. Serve warm.

Nutrition: Calories 246, Total Fat 7.4 g, Saturated Fat 4.6 g, Cholesterol 105 mg, Total Carbs 9.4 g, Sugar 6.5 g, Fiber 2.7 g, Sodium 353 mg, Potassium 529 mg, Protein 37.2 g

Barbeque Chicken Wings

Preparation Time: 10 Minutes Cooking Time: 3 Hours Servings: 4

Ingredients:
- 2 lbs. chicken wings
- 1/2 cup of water
- 1/2 teaspoon of basil, dried
- 3/4 cup of BBQ sauce
- 1/2 cup of lime juice

Directions:
- 1 teaspoon of red pepper, crushed
- 2 teaspoons of paprika
- 1/2 cup of swerve
- Salt and black pepper- to taste
- A pinch cayenne peppers

1. Start by throwing all the Ingredients: into the Slow cooker and mix them well.
2. Cover it and cook for 3 hours on Low Settings.
3. Garnish as desired.
4. Serve warm.

Nutrition: Calories 457, Total Fat 19.1 g, Saturated Fat 11 g, Cholesterol 262 mg, Total Carbs 8.9 g, Sugar 1.2 g, Fiber 1.7 g, Sodium 557 mg, Potassium 748 mg, Protein 32.5 g

Saucy Duck

Preparation Time: 10 Minutes Cooking Time: 6 Hours Servings: 4

Ingredients:
- 1 duck, cut into small chunks
- 4 garlic cloves, minced
- 4 tablespoons of swerves
- 2 green onions, roughly diced
- 4 tablespoon of soy sauce

Directions:
- 4 tablespoon of sherry wine
- 1/4 cup of water
- 1-inch ginger root, sliced
- A pinch salt
- black pepper to taste

1. Start by throwing all the Ingredients: into the Slow cooker and mix them well.
2. Cover it and cook for 6 hours on Low Settings.
3. Garnish as desired.

4. Serve warm.
Nutrition: Calories 338, Total Fat 3.8 g, Saturated Fat 0.7 g, Cholesterol 22 mg, Total Carbs 8.3 g, Fiber 2.4 g, Sugar 1.2 g, Sodium 620 mg, Potassium 271 mg, Protein 15.4g

Chicken Roux Gumbo

Preparation Time: 10 Minutes **Cooking Time:** 6 Hours **Servings:** 24
Ingredients:
- 1 lb. chicken thighs, cut into halves
- 1 tablespoon of vegetable oil
- 1 lb. smoky sausage, sliced, crispy, and crumbled.
- Salt and black pepper- to taste Aromatics:
- 1 bell pepper, diced
- 2 quarts' chicken stock
- 15 oz. canned tomatoes, diced
- 1 celery stalk, diced

Directions:
- salt to taste
- 4 garlic cloves, minced
- 1/2 lbs. okra, sliced
- 1 yellow onion, diced
- a dash tabasco sauce For the roux:
- 1/2 cup of almond flour
- 1/4 cup of vegetable oil
- 1 teaspoon of Cajun spice

1. Start by throwing all the Ingredients: except okra and roux Ingredients: into the Slow cooker.
2. Cover it and cook for 5 hours on Low Settings. Stir in okra and cook for another 1 hour on low heat.
3. Mix all the roux Ingredients: and add them to the Slow cooker.
4. Stir cook on high heat until the sauce thickens.
5. Garnish as desired. Serve warm.

Nutrition: Calories 604, Total Fat 30.6 g, Saturated Fat 13.1 g, Cholesterol 131 mg, Total Carbs 1.4g, Fiber 0.2 g, Sugar 20.3 g, Sodium 834 mg, Potassium 512 mg, Protein 54.6 g

Cider-Braised Chicken

Preparation Time: 10 Minutes **Cooking Time:** 5 Hours **Servings:** 2
Ingredients:
- 4 chicken drumsticks
- 2 tablespoon of olive oil
- ½ cup of apple cider vinegar
- 1 tablespoon of balsamic vinegar

Directions:
- 1 chili pepper, diced
- 1 yellow onion, minced
- Salt and black pepper- to taste

1. Start by throwing all the Ingredients: into a bowl and mix them well.
2. Marinate this chicken for 2 hours in the refrigerator.
3. Spread the chicken along with its marinade in the Slow cooker.
4. Cover it and cook for 5 hours on Low Settings.
5. Garnish as desired. Serve warm.

Nutrition: Calories 311, Total Fat 25.5 g, Saturated Fat 12.4 g, Cholesterol 69 mg, Total Carbs 1.4 g, Fiber 0.7 g, Sugar 0.3 g, Sodium 58 mg, Potassium 362 mg, Protein 18.4 g

Chunky Chicken Salsa

Preparation Time: 10 Minutes Cooking Time: 6 Hours Servings: 2
Ingredients:
- 1 lb. chicken breast, skinless and boneless
- 1 cup of chunky salsa

Directions:
- 3/4 teaspoon of cumin
- A pinch oregano
- Salt and black pepper- to taste

1. Start by throwing all the Ingredients: into the Slow cooker and mix them well.
2. Cover it and cook for 6 hours on Low Settings.
3. Garnish as desired.
4. Serve warm.

Nutrition: Calories 541, Total Fat 34 g, Saturated Fat 8.5 g, Cholesterol 69 mg, Total Carbs 3.4 g, Fiber 1.2 g, Sugar 1 g, Sodium 547 mg, Potassium 467 mg, Protein 20.3 g

Dijon Chicken

Preparation Time: 10 Minutes Cooking Time: 6 Hours Servings: 4
Ingredients:
- 2 lbs. chicken thighs, skinless and boneless
- 3/4 cup of chicken stock
- 1/4 cup of lemon juice

Directions:
- 2 tablespoon of extra virgin olive oil
- 3 tablespoon of Dijon mustard
- 2 tablespoons of Italian seasoning
- Salt and black pepper- to taste

1. Start by throwing all the Ingredients: into the Slow cooker and mix them well.
2. Cover it and cook for 6 hours on Low Settings.
3. Garnish as desired.
4. Serve warm.

Nutrition: Calories 398, Total Fat 13.8 g, Saturated Fat 5.1 g, Cholesterol 200 mg, Total Carbs 3.6 g, Fiber 1 g, Sugar 1.3 g, Sodium 272 mg, Potassium 531 mg, Protein 51.8 g

Chicken Thighs with Vegetables

Preparation Time: 10 Minutes Cooking Time: 6 Hours Servings: 6
Ingredients:
- 6 chicken thighs
- 1 teaspoon of vegetable oil
- 15 oz. canned tomatoes, diced
- 1 yellow onion, diced
- 2 tablespoon of tomato paste
- 1/2 cup of white wine

Directions:
- 2 cups of chicken stock
- 1 celery stalk, diced
- 1/4 lb. baby carrots, cut into halves
- 1/2 teaspoon of thyme, dried
- Salt and black pepper- to taste

1. Start by throwing all the Ingredients: into the Slow cooker and mix them well.
2. Cover it and cook for 6 hours on Low Settings.
3. Shred the slow-cooked chicken using a fork and return to the pot.
4. Mix well and garnish as desired.

5. Serve warm.
Nutrition: Calories 372, Total Fat 11.8 g, Saturated Fat 4.4 g, Cholesterol 62 mg, Total Carbs 1.8 g, Fiber 0.6 g, Sugar 27.3 g, Sodium 871 mg, Potassium 288 mg, Protein 34 g

Chicken Dipped in Tomatillo Sauce

Preparation Time: 10 Minutes Cooking Time: 6 Hours Servings: 4
Ingredients:
- 1 lb. chicken thighs, skinless and boneless
- 2 tablespoon of extra virgin olive oil
- 1 yellow onion, sliced
- 1 garlic clove, crushed
- 4 oz. canned green chilies, diced
- 1 handful cilantro, diced

Directions:
- 15 oz. cauliflower rice, already cooked
- 5 oz. tomatoes, diced
- 15 oz. cheddar cheese, grated
- 4 oz. black olives, pitted and diced
- Salt and black pepper- to taste
- 15 oz canned tomatillos, diced

1. Start by throwing all the Ingredients: into the Slow cooker and mix them well.
2. Cover it and cook for 5 6 hours on Low Settings.
3. Shred the slow-cooked chicken and return to the pot.
4. Mix well and garnish as desired.
5. Serve warm.

Nutrition: Calories 427, Total Fat 31.1 g, Saturated Fat 4.2 g, Cholesterol 0 mg, Total Carbs 9 g, Sugar 12.4 g, Fiber 19.8 g, Sodium 86 mg, Potassium 100 mg, Protein 23.5 g

Chicken with Lemon Parsley Butter

Preparation Time: 10 Minutes Cooking Time: 3 Hours Servings: 10
Ingredients:
- 1 (5 – 6lbs) whole roasting chicken, rinsed
- 1 cup of water
- 1/2 teaspoon of kosher salt
- 1/4 teaspoon of black pepper

Directions:
- 1 whole lemon, sliced
- 4 tablespoons of butter
- 2 tablespoons of fresh parsley, chopped

1. Start by seasoning the chicken with all the herbs and spices.
2. Place this chicken in the Slow cooker.
3. Cover it and cook for 3 hours on High Settings.
4. Meanwhile, melt butter with lemon slices and parsley in a saucepan.
5. Drizzle the butter over the Slow cooker chicken.
6. Serve warm.

Nutrition: Calories 379, Total Fat 29.7 g, Saturated Fat 18.6 g, Cholesterol 141 mg, Total Carbs 9.7g, Fiber 0.9 g, Sugar 1.3 g, Sodium 193 mg, Potassium 131 mg, Protein 25.2 g

Paprika Chicken

Preparation Time: 10 Minutes Cooking Time: 8 Hours Servings: 8
Ingredients:
- 1 free-range whole chicken

- 1 tablespoon of olive oil
- 1 tablespoon of dried paprika

Directions:
- 1 tablespoon of curry powder
- 1 teaspoon of dried turmeric
- 1 teaspoon of salt

1. Start by mixing all the spices and oil in a bowl except chicken.
2. Now season the chicken with these spices liberally.
3. Add the chicken and spices to your Slow cooker.
4. Cover the lid of the slow cooker and cook for 8 hours on Low.
5. Serve warm.

Nutrition: Calories 313, Total Fat 134g, Saturated Fat 78 g, Cholesterol 861 mg, Total Carbs 6.3 g, Fiber 0.7 g, Sugar 19 g, Sodium 62 mg, Potassium 211 mg, Protein 24.6 g

Rotisserie Chicken

Preparation Time: 5 Minutes Cooking Time: 8 Hours
Servings: 8
Ingredients:
- 1 organic whole chicken
- 1 tablespoon of olive oil
- 1 teaspoon of thyme

Directions:
- 1 teaspoon of rosemary
- 1 teaspoon of garlic, granulated
- salt and pepper

1. Start by seasoning the chicken with all the herbs and spices.
2. Broil this seasoned chicken for 5 minutes in the oven until golden brown.
3. Place this chicken in the Slow cooker.
4. Cover it and cook for 8 hours on Low Settings.
5. Serve warm.

Nutrition: Calories 301, Total Fat 12.2 g, Saturated Fat 2.4 g, Cholesterol 110 mg, Total Carbs 2.5 g, Fiber 0.9 g, Sugar 1.4 g, Sodium 276 mg, Potassium 231 mg, Protein 28.8 g

Chicken Ginger Curry

Preparation Time: 10 Minutes Cooking Time: 6 Hours Servings: 4
Ingredients:
- 1 ½ lbs. chicken drumsticks (approx. 5 drumsticks), skin removed
- 1 (13.5 oz.) can coconut milk
- 1 onion, diced
- 4 cloves garlic, minced
- 1-inch knob fresh ginger, minced

Directions:
- 1 Serrano pepper, minced
- 1 tablespoon of Garam Masala
- ½ teaspoon of cayenne
- ½ teaspoon of paprika
- ½ teaspoon of turmeric
- salt and pepper, adjust to taste

1. Start by throwing all the Ingredients: into the Slow cooker.
2. Cover it and cook for 6 hours on Low Settings.
3. Garnish as desired.
4. Serve warm.

Nutrition: Calories 248, Total Fat 15.7 g, Saturated Fat 2.7 g, Cholesterol 75 mg, Total Carbs 8.4 g, Fiber 0g, Sugar 1.1 g, Sodium 94 m, Potassium 331 mg, Protein 14.1 g

Thai Chicken Curry

Preparation Time: 10 Minutes Cooking Time: 2 Hours and 30 Minutes Servings: 2
Ingredients:
- 1 can coconut milk
- 1/2 cup of chicken stock
- 1lb. boneless, skinless chicken thighs, diced
- 1 2 tablespoons of red curry paste
- 1 tablespoon of coconut aminos

Directions:
- 1 tablespoon of fish sauce
- 2 3 garlic cloves, minced
- Salt and black pepper to taste
- red pepper flakes as desired
- 1 bag frozen mixed veggies

1. Start by throwing all the Ingredients: except vegetables into the Slow cooker.
2. Cover it and cook for 2 hours on Low Settings.
3. Remove its lid and thawed veggies.
4. Cover the slow cooker again, then continue cooking for another 30 minutes on Low settings.
5. Garnish as desired.
6. Serve warm.

Nutrition: Calories 327, Total Fat 3.5 g, Saturated Fat 0.5 g, Cholesterol 162 mg, Total Carbs 56g, Fiber 0.4 g, Sugar 0.5 g, Sodium 142 mg, Potassium 558 mg, Protein 21.5 g

CHAPTER 8: MEAT
Mexican Lamb Fillet

Preparation Time: 5 Minutes Cooking Time: 8 Hours
Servings: 4
Ingredients:
- 1 chili pepper, deseeded and chopped
- 1 jalapeno pepper, deseeded and chopped
- 1 cup sweet corn
- 1 cup chicken stock
- 14 oz lamb fillet
- 1 tsp salt

Directions:
- 1 tsp ground black pepper
- 1 tbsp ground paprika
- 1 tsp grated ginger
- 1 cup tomato juice
- 1 tbsp white sugar

1. Add the peppers, ginger, and ground paprika to the blender jug. Blend this peppers mixture for 30 seconds until smooth. Place the lamb fillet to the insert of the Slow cooker.
2. Add pepper mixture, tomato juice, white sugar, black pepper, and salt to the lamb.
3. Lastly, add sweet corn and chicken stock. Put the cooker's lid on and set the cooking time to 8 hours on Low settings.
4. Shred the cooked lamb and return the cooker.
5. Mix well and serve warm.

Nutrition: Calories: 348, Total Fat: 18.3g, Fiber: 3g, Total Carbs: 19.26g, Protein: 28g

Beef Mac & Cheese

Preparation Time: 5 Minutes
Cooking Time: 4 Hours and 30 Minutes Servings: 4
Ingredients:
- ½ cup macaroni, cooked
- 10 oz ground beef - ½ cup marinara sauce

Directions:
- 1 cup Mozzarella, shredded
- ½ cup of water

1. Mix the ground beef with marinara sauce and water and transfer in the Slow cooker.
2. Cook it on High for 4 hours. After this, add macaroni and Mozzarella.
3. Carefully mix the meal and cook it for 30 minutes more on high.

Nutrition: Calories, 25.4g Protein, 12.4g Carbohydrates, 1.2g Fat, 68g Fiber, 63mg Cholesterol, 219mg Sodium, 408mg Potassium.

Beef and Scallions Bowl

Preparation Time: 5 Minutes Cooking Time: 5 Hours
Servings: 4
Ingredients:
- 1 teaspoon chili powder
- 2 oz scallions, chopped
- 1-pound beef stew meat, cubed
- 1 cup corn kernels, frozen

Directions:

- 1 cup of water
- 2 tablespoons tomato paste
- 1 teaspoon minced garlic

1. Mix water with tomato paste and pour the liquid into the Slow cooker.
2. Add chili powder, beef, corn kernels, and minced garlic.
3. Close the lid and cook the meal on high for 5 hours.
4. When the meal is cooked, transfer the mixture to the bowls and top with scallions.

Nutrition: Calories, 36.4g Protein, 10.4g Carbohydrates, 7.7g Fat, 2g Fiber, 101mg Cholesterol, 99mg Sodium, 697mg Potassium.

Balsamic Beef

Preparation Time: 5 Minutes Cooking Time: 9 Hours
Servings: 4
Ingredients:
- 1-pound beef stew meat, cubed
- 1 teaspoon cayenne pepper
- 4 tablespoons balsamic vinegar

Directions:
1. Toss the butter in the skillet and melt it.
- ½ cup of water
- 2 tablespoons butter

2. Then add meat and roast it for minutes per side on medium heat.
3. Transfer the meat with butter in the Slow cooker.
4. Add balsamic vinegar, cayenne pepper, and water.
5. Close the lid and cook the meal on Low for 9 hours.

Nutrition: Calories, 34.5g Protein, 0.4g Carbohydrates, 12.9g Fat, 0.1g Fiber, 117mg Cholesterol, 117mg Sodium, 479mg Potassium.

Simple Pork Chop Casserole

Preparation Time: 5 Minutes Cooking Time: 10 Hours
Servings: 4
Ingredients:
- 4 pork chops, bones removed and cut into bite-sized pieces
- 3 tablespoons minced onion

Directions:
- ½ cup of water
- Salt and pepper to taste
- 1 cup heavy cream

1. Place the pork chop slices, onions, and water in the slow cooker.
2. Season with salt and pepper to taste.
3. Close the lid and cook on low for 10 hours or on high for 8 hours.
4. Halfway through the cooking time, pour in the heavy cream.

Nutrition: Calories per serving: 515; Carbohydrates: 2.5g; Protein: 39.2g; Fat: 34.3g; Sugar: 0g; Sodium: 613mg; Fiber:0.9 g

Balsamic Lamb Chops

Preparation Time: 5 Minutes Cooking Time: 6 Hours Servings: 2
Ingredients:
- 1-pound lamb chops
- 2 tablespoons balsamic vinegar
- 1 tablespoon chives, chopped
- 1 tablespoon olive oil

Directions:
- 4 garlic cloves, minced
- ½ cup beef stock
- A pinch of salt and black pepper

1. In your Slow cooker, mix the lamb chops with the vinegar and the other ingredients, toss, put the lid on and cook on Low for 6 hours.
2. Divide everything between plates and serve.

Nutrition: Calories 292, Fat 12, Fiber 3, Carbs 7, Protein 16

Lamb and Cabbage

Preparation Time: 5 Minutes Cooking Time: 5 Hours
Servings: 2
Ingredients:
- 2 pounds lamb stew meat, cubed
- 1 cup red cabbage, shredded
- 1 cup beef stock
- 1 teaspoon avocado oil

Directions:
- 1 teaspoon sweet paprika
- 2 tablespoons tomato paste
- A pinch of salt and black pepper
- 1 tablespoon cilantro, chopped

1. In your Slow cooker, mix the lamb with the cabbage, stock, and the other ingredients, toss, put the lid on and cook on High for 5 hours.
2. Divide everything between plates and serve.

Nutrition: Calories 254, Fat 12, Fiber 3, Carbs 6, Protein 16

Lavender and Orange Lamb

Preparation Time: 5 Minutes Cooking Time: 7 Hours
Servings: 4
Ingredients:
- 2 tablespoons rosemary, chopped
- 1 and ½ pounds lamb chops
- Salt and black pepper to the taste
- 1 tablespoon lavender, chopped
- 2 garlic cloves, minced

Directions:
- 1 red-orange, cut into halves
- 2 red oranges, peeled and cut into segments
- 2 small pieces of orange peel
- 1 teaspoon butter

1. In a bowl, mix lamb chops with salt, pepper, rosemary, lavender, garlic, and orange peel, toss to coat and leave aside for a couple of hours in the fridge.
2. Put the butter in your Slow cooker, add lamb chops, squeeze one orange over them, add the rest of the oranges over the lamb, cover the Slow cooker and cook on Low for 7 hours.
3. Divide lamb and sauce all over and serve.

Nutrition: Calories 250, Fat 5, Fiber 7, Carbs 15, Protein 20

Beer Sausages

Preparation Time: 5 Minutes Cooking Time: 7 Hours
Servings: 4
Ingredients:
- 1-pound beef sausages
- 3 tablespoons butter
- 1 teaspoon ground black pepper

Directions:
1. Toss the butter in the skillet and melt it.
- 1 teaspoon salt
- 1 cup beer
2. Add beef sausages and roast them on high heat for minutes per side.
3. Transfer the beef sausages to the Slow cooker.
4. Add ground black pepper, salt, and beer.
5. Close the lid and cook the meal on Low for 7 hours.

Nutrition: Calories 304, Fat 24.9, Fiber 5.4, Carbs 6.5, Protein 13.8

Hamburger Style Stuffing

Preparation Time: 5 Minutes Cooking Time: 3 Hours
Servings: 4
Ingredients:
- 1-pound ground pork
- ½ cup Cheddar cheese, shredded
- ½ cup fresh cilantro, chopped
- ¼ cup onion, minced

Directions:
- 1 cup of water
- ¼ cup tomato juice
- 1 bell pepper, diced
- 1 teaspoon salt

1. Mix ground pork with cilantro, onion, and diced pepper.
2. Then transfer the mixture to the Slow cooker.
3. Add all remaining ingredients and mix.
4. Close the lid and cook the stuffing on High for 3 hours.

Nutrition: 235 Calories, 33.7g Protein, 3.8g Carbohydrates, 8.8g Fat, 0.7g Fiber, 98mg Cholesterol, 778mg Sodium, 604mg Potassium

Classic Pork Adobo

Preparation Time: 5 Minutes Cooking Time: 12 Hours
Servings: 6
Ingredients:
- 2 pounds pork chops, sliced
- 4 cloves of garlic, minced
- 1 onion, chopped
- 2 bay leaves

Directions:
- ¼ cup of soy sauce
- ½ cup lemon juice, freshly squeezed
- 4 quail eggs, boiled and peeled

1. Place all ingredients except the quail eggs in the Slow cooker.
2. Give a good stir.
3. Close the lid and cook on high for 10 hours or on low for 12 hours.
4. Add in quail eggs an hour before the cooking time ends.

Nutrition: Calories per serving: 371; Carbohydrates: 6.4g; Protein: 40.7g; Fat: 24.1g; Sugar: 0g; Sodium: 720mg; Fiber: 3.9g

Pork Ragu With Basil

Preparation Time: 5 Minutes **Cooking Time:** 4 Hours
Servings: 4
Ingredients:
- 8 oz pork loin, chopped
- 1 cup russet potatoes
- ½ cup carrot, chopped
- 3 oz fennel bulb, chopped
- 1 tablespoon dried basil

Directions:
- 1 teaspoon salt
- 3 cups of water
- ½ cup plain yogurt
- 1 teaspoon tomato paste

1. In the mixing bowl, mix tomato paste with plain yogurt, salt, dried basil, and pork loin.
2. Transfer the mixture to the Slow cooker and close the lid.
3. Cook the meat on high for 2 hours.
4. Then add water and all remaining ingredients. Carefully mix the mixture.
5. Close the lid and cook the ragu on low for hours.

Nutrition: 198 Calories, 18.3g Protein, 11.2g Carbohydrates, 8.4g Fat, 2g Fiber, 47mg Cholesterol, 667mg Sodium, 613mg Potassium

Indian Style Cardamom Pork

Preparation Time: 5 Minutes **Cooking Time:** 6 Hours
Servings: 4
Ingredients:
- 1-pound pork steak, tenderized
- 1 teaspoon ground cardamom
- ½ cup of coconut milk
- 1 teaspoon chili powder

Directions:
- 1 teaspoon ground turmeric
- 1 teaspoon cashew butter
- ¼ cup of water

1. Cut the pork steak into 4 servings and rub with ground cardamom, chili powder. And ground turmeric.
2. Place the meat in the Slow cooker.
3. Add cashew butter, water, and coconut milk.
4. Close the lid and cook the pork on high for 6 hours.

Nutrition: 295 Calories, 21g Protein, 7.2g Carbohydrates, 21.1g Fat, 1.9g Fiber, 69mg Cholesterol, 569mg Sodium, 118mg Potassium

Beef with Spinach

Preparation Time: 5 Minutes **Cooking Time:** 7 Hours
Servings: 2
Ingredients:
- 1 red onion, sliced
- 1-pound beef stew meat, cubed
- 1 cup tomato passata
- 1 cup baby spinach

Directions:
- 1 teaspoon olive oil
- Salt and black pepper to the taste
- ½ cup bee stock
- 1 tablespoon basil, chopped

1. In your Slow cooker, mix the beef with the onion, passata, and the other ingredients except for the spinach, toss, put the lid on and cook on Low for 6 hours and 30 minutes.
2. Add the spinach, toss, put the lid on, cook on Low for 30 minutes more, divide into bowls, and serve.

Nutrition: Calories 400, Fat 15, Fiber 4, Carbs 25, Protein 14

Beef with Peas and Corn

Preparation Time: 5 Minutes **Cooking Time:** 7 Hours
Servings: 2
Ingredients:
- 1-pound beef stew meat, cubed
- ½ cup of corn
- ½ cup fresh peas
- 2 scallions, chopped

Directions:
- 1 tablespoon lime juice
- 1 cup beef stock
- 2 tablespoons tomato paste
- ½ cup chives, chopped

1. In your Slow cooker, mix the beef with the corn, peas, and the other ingredients, toss, put the lid on and cook on Low for 7 hours.
2. Divide the mix between plates and serve right away.

Nutrition: Calories 236, Fat 12, Fiber 2, Carbs 7, Protein 15

Barbacoa Lamb

Preparation Time: 5 Minutes **Cooking Time:** 6 Hours
Servings: 12
Ingredients:
- ¼ c. dried mustard
- 5 ½ lbs. leg of lamb - boneless
- 2 tbsp. of each: Smoked paprika and Himalayan salt

Directions:
- 1 tbsp. of each: Chipotle powder, Dried oregano, Ground cumin
- 1 c. water

1. Combine the paprika, oregano, chipotle powder, cumin, and salt.
2. Cover the roast with the dried mustard, and sprinkle with the prepared spices. Arrange the lamb in the slow cooker, cover, and let it marinate in the refrigerator overnight.
3. In the morning, let the pot come to room temperature. Once you're ready to cook, just add the cup of water to the slow cooker on the high heat setting. Cook for six hours.
4. When done, remove all except for one cup of the cooking juices, and shred the lamb.
5. Using the rest of the cooking juices - adjust the seasoning as you desire, and serve

Nutrition: 492 Calories, 1.2 g Net Carbs, 35.8 g Fat, 37.5 g Protein

Lamb with Mint & Green Beans

Preparation Time: 5 Minutes **Cooking Time:** 6 to 10 Hours
Servings: 4
Ingredients:
- ½ t. salt – Himalayan pink

- Freshly cracked black pepper
- 1 lamb leg – bone-in
- 2 tbsp. lard/ghee/tallow

Directions:
1. Heat the slow cooker with the high setting.
- 4 garlic cloves
- 6 c. trimmed green beans
- ¼ freshly chopped mint/1-2 tbsp. dried mint

2. Dry the lamb with some paper towels. Sprinkle with the pepper and salt. Grease a Dutch oven or similar large pot with the ghee/lard.
3. Sear the lamb until golden brown and set aside.
4. Remove the peels from the garlic and mince. Dice up the mint. Arrange the seared meat into the slow cooker and give it a shake of the garlic and mint.
5. Secure the lid and program the cooker on the low-heat function (10 hrs.) or the high-function (6 hrs.).
6. After about four hours, switch the lamb out of the cooker. Toss in the green beans and return the lamb back into the pot. Note: You can add ½ cup to one cup of water to the cooker if it gets dried out.
7. Let the flavors mingle for about two more hours. The meat should be tender and the beans crispy. Serve and enjoy!

Nutrition: 525 Calories, 7.6 g Net Carb, 37.3 g Protein, 36.4 g Fat

Succulent Lamb

Preparation Time: 5 Minutes **Cooking Time:** 8 Hours 20 Minutes
Servings: 6
Ingredients:
- ¼ c. olive oil
- 1 (2 lb.) leg of lamb
- 1 tbsp. maple syrup
- 2 tbsp. whole grain mustard

Directions:
- 4 thyme sprigs
- 6-7 mint leaves
- ¾ t. of each: Dried rosemary and Garlic
- Pepper & salt to taste

1. Cut away the string/netting off the lamb. Slice three slits over the top.
2. Cover the meat with the oil and the rub (mustard, pepper, salt, and maple syrup). Push the rosemary and garlic into the slits.
3. Prepare on the low setting for seven hours. Garnish with the mint and thyme. Cook one more hour. Place on a platter and serve.

Nutrition: 414 Calories, 0.3 g Net Carbs, 35.2 g Fats, 26.7 g Protein

Tarragon Lamb & Beans

Preparation Time: 5 Minutes
Cooking Time: 9 Hours and 15 Minutes Servings: 12
Ingredients:
- 4 (1 ½ lb.) lamb shanks
- 1 can (19 0z.) white beans/cannellini- for example - 1 ½ c. peeled - diced carrot
- 2 thinly sliced garlic cloves - 1 c. onion
- ¾ c. celery - 2 t. dried tarragon

Directions:
- ¼ t. freshly cracked black pepper
- 2 t. dried tarragon
- 1 can (28 oz.) diced tomatoes - not drained

- Recommended: 7-quart slow cooker

1. Discard all the fat from the lamb shanks. Pour the beans, cloves of garlic, chopped carrots, chopped celery, and onion into the cooker. Arrange the shanks on top of the beans, and sprinkle with the salt, pepper, and tarragon. Empty the tomatoes over the lamb - including the juices. Cover and cook the lamb on high for approximately one hour. Reduce the temperature to the low setting and cook for nine hours or until the lamb is tender. Take the lamb out of the slow cooker and set it aside. Empty the bean mixture through a colander over a bowl to reserve the liquid. Let the juices stand for five minutes and skim off the fat from the surface.

2. Return the bean mixture to the liquid in the slow cooker. Strip the lamb bones and throw the bones away. Serve with the bean mixture and enjoy yourself with your family and friends.

Nutrition: 353 Calories, 12.9 g Net Carbs, 16.3 g Fat, 50.3 g Protein

BBQ Beef Burritos

Preparation Time: 5 Minutes
Cooking Time: 8 Hours and 15 Minutes Servings: 4
Ingredients:
- 2 lb. top sirloin steak
- ½ t. black pepper
- 1 t. of each: Ground chipotle pepper (optional), Cinnamon
- 2 t. of each: Sea salt, Garlic powder
- 4 minced garlic cloves
- ½ white onion - 2 bay leaves

Directions:
- 1 c. of each: Chicken broth, BBQ sauce –

your favorite Assembly Ingredients
- 1 ½ c. coleslaw mix
- 8 low-carb wraps
- ½ c. mayonnaise

1. Pat the steak dry using some paper towels. Score with a sharp knife along the sides. Combine the seasonings and sprinkle on the meat. Roughly chop the onion and mince the garlic and add to the slow cooker. Pour in the broth. Add the steak and bay leaf. Secure the lid and cook eight hours on the low setting

2. When done, remove the steak and drain the juices. Arrange the beef, garlic, and onion back into the cooker and shred. Pour in the barbecue sauce and mix well. Assemble the burritos using the beef fixings, a bit of slaw, and a dab of mayo.

Nutrition: 750 Calories, 14 g Net Carbs, 48 g Fat, 58 g Protein

Cheeseburger & Bacon Pie

Preparation Time: 5 Minutes Cooking Time: 4 Hours
Servings: 8
Ingredients:
- 6 bacon slices – chopped
- 1 lb. ground beef
- 2 minced garlic cloves
- ¼ t. hot pepper flakes - Pepper & Salt
- 6 large eggs

Directions:
- 4 oz. softened cream cheese
- 1½ c. Mexican shredded cheese/shredded cheese
- Suggested to Use: 6-quart slow cooker

1. Grease the cooker insert about 1/3 of the way up the sides.
2. Prepare the bacon until crispy in a skillet and drain on paper towels. Save the drippings and add the ground beef - cooking (med. heat) until browned.

3. Stir in the pepper flakes, garlic, pepper, and salt. Cook one minute and spread over the bottom of the cooker. Add ¾ of the bacon pieces and one cup of the cheese.
4. Whisk the eggs and cream cheese together until smooth. Scrape over the beef.
5. Prepare 3 ½ to 4 hours using the low-heat setting. The center should be just set.
6. Garnish with the rest of the cheese and secure the lid. Give it ten minutes to melt the cheese and sprinkle with the rest of the bacon. Serve and enjoy!
Nutrition: 376 Calories, 25.93 g Fat, 1.48 g, Net Carbs, 28.21 g Protein

Italian Meatballs & Zoodles

Preparation Time: 5 Minutes
Cooking Time: 6 Hours and 35 Minutes Servings: 12
Ingredients:
- 1 med. spiraled zucchini
- 32. oz. beef stock - 1 small diced onion
- 2 chopped celery ribs
- 1 chopped carrot - 1 med. diced tomato
- 6 minced garlic cloves
- 1 ½ lb. ground beef - 1 ½ t. garlic salt
- ½ c. shredded parmesan cheese

Directions:
1. Heat the slow cooker with the low setting function.
- 1 large egg
- ½ t. black pepper
- 4 tbsp. freshly chopped parsley
- 1 ½ t. of each: (Onion powder Sea salt)
- 1 t. of each: Italian seasoning, and Dried oregano

2. Add the zucchini, beef stock, onion, celery, tomato, garlic salt, and carrot to the cooker. Cover with the lid. Combine the beef, egg, parmesan, parsley, Italian seasonings, pepper, sea salt, oregano, garlic, and onion powder in a mixing container. Mix and shape into 30 meatballs.
3. Warm up the oil using med-high heat in a frying pan. When it's hot, add the meatballs. Brown and toss into the cooker. Prepare with the lid on for six hours on the low setting.
Nutrition: 129 Calories, 3 g Net Carbs, 6 g Fat, 15 g Protein

Italian Meatloaf

Preparation Time: 15 Minutes Cooking Time: 3 Hours Servings: 8
Ingredients:
- 2 lb. ground sirloin - extra-lean
- Non-stick cooking spray/spritzer bottle with olive oil
- 2 large eggs
- 1 c. grated zucchini – approx. 1 medium
- 4 minced garlic cloves
- 1 tbsp. dried oregano
- ½ c. fresh each of: Finely chopped parsley (+) more for topping Grated parmesan cheese
- 3 tbsp. balsamic vinegar

Directions:
- 2 tbsp. onion powder/minced dry onion
- ½ t. of each: Sea salt & ground black pepper

Topping Ingredients
- 2 tbsp. freshly chopped parsley
- ¼ c. of each: Shredded mozzarella cheese

– approx. 2-3 slices
- -Tomato sauce/ketchup

- Suggested for Use: 6-quart oval slow cook

1. Line the cooker with aluminum foil strips, and spray with the cooking spray.
2. Combine all the fixings (leave out the topping ingredients). The mixture will be loose. Shape it into an oblong loaf and arrange on a sling. Make the sling using aluminum foil strips long enough to wrap around the dish to remove it from the slow cooker.
3. Secure the lid. Program the cooker on high (3 hrs.) or low (6 hrs.). Approximately 15 minutes before the end of the cooking cycle, unplug the cooker. Remove the lid and add the toppings.
4. Let the meal rest for another five to ten minutes.
5. Remove it from the pot using the aluminum strips. Then add to a serving platter and sprinkle with some parsley.

Nutrition: 292 Calories, 5 g Net Carbs, 17 g Fat, 29 g Protein

Beef Bourguignon with Carrot Noodles

Preparation Time: 20 Minutes Cooking Time: 5 Hours Servings: 6

Ingredients:
- 5 slices - thick-cut bacon
- 1 (3 lb.) chuck roast/round roast/your favorite
- 1 large yellow onion
- 3 diced celery stalks
- 3 large minced garlic cloves
- 1 bay leaf
- 4 sprigs of fresh thyme
- 1 lb. white button mushrooms - sliced
- 1 tbsp. tomato paste
- 1 c. of each: Beef/chicken broth (+) more as needed and Red wine
- 1 large/2 med. carrots For the Garnish: Chopped parsley
- Salt & Pepper
- Optional: Dash of red pepper flakes

Directions:

1. Prepare the bacon in a frying pan using the med-high setting on the stovetop. Place on a paper towel to drain the grease.
2. Flavor the beef cubes with pepper and salt to taste. Layer the meat in the skillet, and sear for one to three minutes. Flip it over and sear another two to three minutes. Toss it in the slow cooker after all of the cubes are cooked.
3. Fold in the bacon, garlic, mushrooms, celery, and onion in the cooker. Push the thyme and bay leaves between the layers.
4. Empty the broth and wine to cover the mixture (approximately ¾ of the way up the cooker).
5. Close the top and cook for four hours on high. Shred the carrots to make 'noodles' using a peeler). Cover and cook for another hour or until the beef falls from the bone.
6. Trash the bay leaves when the meal is done and mix well.
7. Serve with the parsley and pepper flakes.

Nutrition: 548 Calories, 6 g Net Carbs, 32 g Fat, 50 g Protein

Beef & Broccoli

Preparation Time: 5 Minutes
Cooking Time: 6 Hours and 30 Minutes Servings: 4

Ingredients:
- 2/3 c. liquid aminos
- 2 lbs. flank steak
- 1 c/ beef broth
- 1 t. freshly grated ginger
- 3 tbsp. sweetener - your choice

Directions:
1. Warm up the slow cooker using the low setting.
2. Slice the steak into one to two-inch chunks.
- 3 minced garlic cloves
- ½ t. of each: Salt and Red pepper flakes - to taste - more or less
- 1 head broccoli
- 1 red bell pepper

3. Pour in the beef broth, aminos, and steak - along with the ginger, sweetener, garlic cloves, salt, and red pepper flakes. Cook five to six hours on the low setting.
4. Slice the red pepper into one-inch pieces, and chop the broccoli into florets. After the steak is cooked, stir well. Toss in the peppers and broccoli on top of everything in the slow cooker.
5. Continue cooking for at least one more hour. Add everything together, and sprinkle with sesame seeds for the topping.

Nutrition: 430 Calories, 3 g Net Carbs, 54 g Protein, 19 g Fat

Beef Ribs

Preparation Time: 5 Minutes
Cooking Time: 6 Hours and 30 Minutes Servings: 4
Ingredients:
- 3 lb. beef back ribs
- 1 tbsp. of each: Sesame oil, Rice vinegar, Hot sauce, Garlic powder, and Kosher salt

Directions:
- ½ t. black pepper
- 1 tbsp. potato starch/ cornstarch
- ¼ c. light soy sauce or 1/8 c. coconut aminos

1. Cut and add the ribs to fit in the slow cooker. Whisk the rest of the ingredients together but omit the cornstarch for now. Pour the mixture over the ribs, making sure the sauce covers all sides.
2. Use the low setting and cook for six hours. It will be fall off the bone tender.
3. Prepare the oven to 200ºF.
4. Transfer the prepared ribs to a baking pan, and cover.
5. Use a strainer to pour the liquid from the slow cooker into a saucepan. Prepare on the high setting and whisk in the cornstarch with a little bit of cold water. Continue cooking - whisking often - just until the sauce has thickened into a glaze - usually about five to ten minutes.
6. Brush the glaze over the ribs and serve

Nutrition: 342 Calories, 27 g Fat, 7 g Net Carbs, 23 g Protein

Braised Oxtails

Preparation Time: 5 Minutes Cooking Time: 6 to 7 Hours
Servings: 3
Ingredients:
- 2 c. beef broth
- 2 lbs. (bone-in) oxtails
- 1 tbsp. fish sauce
- 1/3 c. butter
- 2 tbsp. soy sauce
- 1 t of each: Minced garlic, Onion powder, and Dried thyme

Directions:
- 3 tbsp. tomato paste
- Pepper & Salt to taste
- ½ t. guar gum
- ½ t. ground ginger

1. On the stovetop, warm up the broth and combine with the fish sauce, soy sauce, butter, and tomato paste. Pour into the cooker along with the meat and flavor with the spices.
2. Prepare for six to seven hours on the low setting
3. Remove the oxtail and set aside on towels to drain.
4. Add the guar gum to the rest of the liquids and blend to thicken. (An immersion blender is best.)
5. Enjoy with your favorite side dish.
Nutrition: 433 Calories, 3.2 g Net Carbs, 29.7 g Fat, 28.3 g Protein

Brisket & Onions

Preparation Time: 5 Minutes Cooking Time: 6 to 8 Hours
Servings: 6
Ingredients:
- 1 ½ lb. red/yellow onions -2 larges
- 1 tbsp. olive oil
- 3 ½ lb. beef brisket
- 6 minced garlic cloves
- Coarse kosher salt

Directions:
- Freshly cracked black pepper
- 1 tbsp. soy sauce
- 2 c. beef broth
- 2 tbsp. Worcestershire sauce – homemade

1. Prepare a cast iron skillet with the oil (med heat). Slice the onions into half-moons and add them to the pan. Sauté for about 20 minutes until they are lightly caramelized.
2. Pat the brisket dry and season with pepper and salt. Sear until it's crusty brown. Add to the cooker with the fat side up.
3. Add the garlic over the meat along with the lightly browned onions.
4. Prepare the broth (soy, Worcestershire, and broth). Pour it into the slow cooker. Secure the lid and prepare for six to eight hours on the low heat function.
5. Set the cooker to warm when done and let it rest at least 20 minutes or place it in a warm oven in a baking dish. Slice and serve.
Nutrition: 777 Calories, 61.3 g Fat, 4.7 g Net Carbs, 48 g Protein

Italian Ragu

Preparation Time: 5 Minutes Cooking Time: 8 hours Servings: 2
Ingredients:
- ¼ of each - diced: Carrot, Rib of celery, and Onion
- 1 minced garlic clove
- ½ lb. top-round lean beef
- 6 tbsp. (3 oz.) of each: Diced tomatoes and Crushed tomatoes

Directions:
- 2 ½ t. beef broth (+) ¼ c.
- 1 ¼ t. of each: Chopped fresh thyme and Minced fresh rosemary
- 1 bay leaf
- Pepper & Salt to taste

1. Arrange the prepared celery, onion, garlic, and carrots into the slow cooker. Trim away the fat, and toss in the meat. Sprinkle with the salt and pepper
2. Stir in the rest of the fixings. Prepare on the low setting for six to eight hours.
3. Enjoy any way you choose.
Nutrition: 224 Calories, 6 g Net Carbs, 27 g Protein, 9 g Fat

Mississippi Pot Roast

Preparation Time: 15 Minutes Cooking Time: 8 Hours Servings: 8
Ingredients:
- 1 jar (16 oz.) deli-sliced pepperoncini
- 1 (3.8 lbs.) beef chuck roast
- ½ t. salt
- 1 tbsp. of each: Dried chives, Dried dill, Onion powder, Dried parsley, and Garlic powder

Directions:
1. Drain the pepperoncini and reserve the brine.
- ¼ t. black pepper
- 2 tbsp. Better than Bouillon

2. Program the slow cooker using the high setting. Add the roast and pepperoncini. Pour one cup of the brine into the cooker and throw away the rest of the liquid. Stir in the bouillon paste and spices. Lastly, add the stick of butter. Prepare using the high setting for eight to ten hours. You don't need to stir.

3. When the roast is done, just shred it with a fork and serve.

Nutrition: 435.22 Calories, 3.13 g Net Carbs, 31.64 g Fat, 33.21 g Protein

CHAPTER 9: VEGETABLE MEALS

Aloo Gobi

Preparation Time: 15 Minutes - Cooking Time: 5 Hours Servings: 4
Ingredients:
- 1 large cauliflower, cut into 1-inch pieces
- 1 large russet potato, peeled and diced
- 1 medium yellow onion, peeled and diced
- 1 cup canned diced tomatoes, with juice
- 1 cup frozen peas - ¼ cup of water
- 1 (2-inch) piece fresh ginger, peeled and finely chopped

Directions:
- 1½ teaspoons minced garlic (3 cloves)
- 1 jalapeño pepper, stemmed and sliced
- 1 tablespoon cumin seeds
- 1 tablespoon garam masala
- 1 teaspoon ground turmeric
- 1 heaping tablespoon fresh cilantro
- Cooked rice, for serving (optional)

1. Combine the cauliflower, potato, onion, diced tomatoes, peas, water, ginger, garlic, jalapeño, cumin seeds, garam masala, and turmeric in a slow cooker; mix until well combined.
2. Cover and cook on low for 4 to 5 hours. Garnish with the cilantro, and serve over cooked rice (if using).

Nutrition: Calories: 115; Total fat: <1g; Protein: 6g; Sodium: 62mg; Fiber: 6g

Jackfruit Carnitas

Preparation Time: 15 Minutes - Cooking Time: 8 Hours - Servings: 4
Ingredients:
- 2 (20-ounce) cans jackfruit, drained, hard pieces discarded
- ¾ cup Very Easy Vegetable Broth or store-bought - 1 tablespoon ground cumin
- 1 tablespoon dried oregano
- 1½ teaspoons ground coriander

Directions:
- 1 teaspoon minced garlic (2 cloves)
- ½ teaspoon ground cinnamon
- 2 bay leaves - Tortillas, for serving
- Optional toppings: diced onions, sliced radishes, fresh cilantro, lime wedges, Nacho Cheese

1. Combine the jackfruit, vegetable broth, cumin, oregano, coriander, garlic, cinnamon, and bay leaves in a slow cooker. Stir to combine. Cover and cook on low for 8 hours or on high for 4 hours.
2. Use two forks to pull the jackfruit apart into shreds.
3. Remove the bay leaves. Serve in warmed tortillas with your favorite taco fixings.

Nutrition: Calories: 286; Total fat: 2g; Protein: 6g; Sodium: 155mg; Fiber: 5g

Baked Beans

Preparation Time: 15 Minutes Cooking Time: 6 Hours Servings: 4
Ingredients:
- 2 (15-ounce) cans white beans, drained and rinsed
- 1 (15-ounce) can tomato sauce
- 1 medium yellow onion, finely diced
- 1½ teaspoons minced garlic (3 cloves)
- 3 tablespoons brown sugar

Directions:

- 2 tablespoons molasses
- 1 tablespoon prepared yellow mustard
- 1 tablespoon chili powder
- 1 teaspoon soy sauce
- Pinch salt
- Freshly ground black pepper

1. Place the beans, tomato sauce, onion, garlic, brown sugar, molasses, mustard, chili powder, and soy sauce into a slow cooker; mix well.
2. Cover and cook on low for 6 hours. Season with salt and pepper before serving.

Nutrition: Calories: 468; Total fat: 2g; Protein: 28g; Sodium: 714mg; Fiber: 20g

Brussels Sprouts Curry

Preparation Time: 15 Minutes Cooking Time: 8 Hours Servings: 4
Ingredients:
- ¾ pound Brussels sprouts, bottoms cut off and sliced in half
- 1 can full-fat coconut milk
- 1 cup Very Easy Vegetable Broth or store-bought
- 1 medium onion, diced
- 1 medium carrot, thinly sliced
- 1 medium red or Yukon potato, diced
- 1½ teaspoons minced garlic (3 cloves)
- 1 (1-inch) piece fresh ginger, peeled and minced

Directions:
- 1 small serrano chile, seeded and finely chopped
- 2 tablespoons peanut butter
- 1 tablespoon rice vinegar or other vinegar
- 1 tablespoon cane sugar or agave nectar
- 1 tablespoon soy sauce
- 1 teaspoon curry powder
- 1 teaspoon ground turmeric
- Pinch salt
- Freshly ground black pepper
- Cooked rice, for serving (optional)

1. Place the Brussels sprouts, coconut milk, vegetable broth, onion, carrot, potato, garlic, ginger, serrano chile, peanut butter, vinegar, cane sugar, soy sauce, curry powder, and turmeric in a slow cooker. Mix well.
2. Cover and cook on low for 7 to 8 hours or on high for 4 to 5 hours.
3. Season with salt and pepper. Serve over rice (if using).

Nutrition: Calories: 404; Total fat: 29g; Protein: 10g; Sodium: 544mg; Fiber: 8g

Jambalaya

Preparation Time: 15 Minutes Cooking Time: 8 Hours Servings: 4
Ingredients:
- 2 cups Very Easy Vegetable Broth or store-bought
- 1 large yellow onion, diced
- 1 green bell pepper, seeded and chopped
- 2 celery stalks, chopped
- 1½ teaspoons minced garlic (3 cloves)
- 1 (15-ounce) can dark red kidney beans, drained and rinsed
- 1 (15-ounce) can black-eyed peas, drained and rinsed

Directions:
- 1 (15-ounce) can diced tomatoes, drained
- 2 tablespoons Cajun seasoning

- 2 teaspoons dried oregano
- 2 teaspoons dried parsley
- 1 teaspoon cayenne pepper
- 1 teaspoon smoked paprika
- ½ teaspoon dried thyme
- Cooked rice, for serving (optional)

1. Combine the vegetable broth, onion, bell pepper, celery, garlic, kidney beans, black-eyed peas, diced tomatoes, Cajun seasoning, oregano, parsley, cayenne pepper, smoked paprika, and dried thyme in a slow cooker; mix well.
2. Cover and cook on low for 6 to 8 hours.
3. Serve over rice (if using).

Nutrition: Calories: 428; Total fat: 2g; Protein: 28g; Sodium: 484mg; Fiber: 19g

Mushroom-Kale Stroganoff

Preparation Time: 15 Minutes Cooking Time: 8 Hours
Servings: 4
Ingredients:
- 1-pound mushrooms, sliced
- 1½ cups Very Easy Vegetable Broth or store-bought
- 1 cup stemmed and chopped kale
- 1 small yellow onion, diced
- 2 garlic cloves, minced

Directions:
- 2 tablespoons all-purpose flour
- 2 tablespoons ketchup or tomato paste
- 2 teaspoons paprika
- ½ cup vegan sour cream
- ¼ cup chopped fresh parsley
- Cooked rice, pasta, or quinoa, for serving

1. Combine the mushrooms, vegetable broth, kale, onion, garlic, flour, ketchup or tomato paste, and paprika in a slow cooker. Mix thoroughly.
2. Cover and cook on low for 6 to 8 hours.
3. Stir in the sour cream and parsley just before serving.
4. Serve over rice, pasta, or quinoa.

Nutrition: Calories: 146; Total fat: 7g; Protein: 8g; Sodium: 417mg; Fiber: 3g

Sloppy Joe Filling

Preparation Time: 15 Minutes Cooking Time: 8 Hours Servings: 4
Ingredients:
- 3 cups textured vegetable protein
- 3 cups of water
- 2 (6-ounce) cans tomato paste or 1 cup ketchup
- 1 medium yellow onion, diced
- ½ medium green bell pepper, finely diced
- 2 teaspoons minced garlic (4 cloves)
- 4 tablespoons vegan Worcestershire sauce

Directions:
- 3 tablespoons brown sugar
- 3 tablespoons apple cider vinegar
- 3 tablespoons prepared yellow mustard
- 2 tablespoons hot sauce (optional)
- 1 tablespoon salt
- 1 teaspoon chili powder

- Sliced, toasted buns or cooked rice, for serving

1. Combine the textured vegetable protein, water, tomato paste, onion, bell pepper, garlic, Worcestershire sauce, brown sugar, vinegar, mustard, hot sauce (if using), salt, and chili powder in a slow cooker. Mix well.
2. Cover and cook on low for 6 to 8 hours or on high for 4 to 5 hours.
3. Serve on sliced, toasted buns or over rice.

Nutrition: Calories: 452; Total fat: 4g; Protein: 75g; Sodium: 2,242mg; Fiber: 11g

Hoppin' John

Preparation Time: 15 Minutes Cooking Time: 6 Hours Servings: 4
Ingredients:
- 3 (15-ounce) cans black-eyed peas, drained and rinsed
- 1 (14.5-ounce) can Cajun-style stewed tomatoes, with juice
- 2 cups hot water
- 1 cup stemmed and chopped kale
- ¾ cup finely diced red bell pepper

Directions:
- ½ cup sliced scallions
- 1 medium jalapeño pepper, seeded and minced
- 1 teaspoon minced garlic (2 cloves)
- 1½ teaspoons hot sauce
- 1 vegetable bouillon cube
- Cooked rice, for serving

1. Combine the black-eyed peas, tomatoes, hot water, kale, bell pepper, scallions, jalapeño, garlic, hot sauce, and bouillon cube in a slow cooker. Stir to combine.
2. Cover and cook on low for 4 to 6 hours.
3. Serve over cooked rice.

Nutrition: Calories: 164; Total fat: 2g; Protein: 10g; Sodium: 250mg; Fiber: 8g

African Sweet Potato Stew

Preparation Time: 15 Minutes Cooking Time: 8 Hours Servings: 4
Ingredients:
- 4 cups peeled diced sweet potatoes
- 1 (15-ounce) can red kidney beans, drained and rinsed
- 1 (14.5-ounce) can diced tomatoes, drained
- 1 cup diced red bell pepper
- 2 cups Very Easy Vegetable Broth or store-bought

Directions:
- 1 medium yellow onion, chopped
- 1 (4.5-ounce) can chopped green chiles, drained
- 1 teaspoon minced garlic (2 cloves)
- 1½ teaspoons ground ginger
- 1 teaspoon ground cumin
- 4 tablespoons creamy peanut butter
- Pinch salt - Freshly ground black pepper

1. Combine the sweet potatoes, kidney beans, diced tomatoes, bell pepper, vegetable broth, onion, green chiles, garlic, ginger, and cumin in a slow cooker. Mix well.
2. Cover and cook on low for 7 to 8 hours.
3. Spoon a little of the soup into a small bowl and mix in the peanut butter, then pour the mixture back into the stew. Season with salt and pepper. Mix well and serve.

Nutrition: Calories: 514; Total fat: 10g; Protein: 22g; Sodium: 649mg; Fiber: 17g

Sweet-and-Sour Tempeh

Preparation Time: 15 Minutes Cooking Time: 8 Hours Servings: 4
Ingredients:
FOR THE SAUCE
- ¾ cup fresh or canned pineapple chunks
- ½ cup crushed tomatoes
- ½ cup of water - ¼ cup chopped onion
- ¼ cup of soy sauce
- 2 tablespoons rice vinegar
- ¼ teaspoon red pepper flakes

Directions:
TO MAKE THE SAUCE
- 1 (½-inch) piece fresh ginger, peeled FOR THE TEMPEH
- 2 (8-ounce) packages tempeh, cut into cubes - 2 cups diced bell pepper
- 1½ cups diced pineapple
- ½ cup diced onion
- Cooked rice, for serving

1. Put the pineapple chunks, crushed tomatoes, water, onion, soy sauce, rice vinegar, red pepper flakes, and ginger in a blender; blend until smooth.
TO MAKE THE TEMPEH
2. Combine the sauce, tempeh, bell pepper, diced pineapple, and onion in a slow cooker; stir well.
3. Cover and cook on low for 7 to 8 hours. Serve over cooked rice.
Nutrition: Calories: 324; Total fat: 13g; Protein: 24g; Sodium: 974mg; Fiber: 4g

Delightful Dal

Preparation Time: 15 Minutes Cooking Time: 7 Hours Servings: 4
Ingredients:
- 3 cups red lentils, rinsed
- 6 cups water
- 1 (28-ounce) can diced tomatoes, with juice
- 1 small yellow onion, diced
- 2½ teaspoons minced garlic (5 cloves)
- 1 (1-inch) piece fresh ginger, peeled and minced
- 1 tablespoon ground turmeric

Directions:
- 2 teaspoons ground cumin
- 1½ teaspoons ground cardamom
- 1½ teaspoons whole mustard seeds
- 1 teaspoon fennel seeds
- 1 bay leaf
- 1 teaspoon salt
- ¼ teaspoon freshly ground black pepper

1. Combine the lentils, water, diced tomatoes, onion, garlic, ginger, turmeric, cumin, cardamom, mustard seeds, fennel seeds, bay leaf, salt, and pepper in a slow cooker; mix well.
2. Cover and cook on low for 7 to 9 hours or on high for 4 to 6 hours. Remove the bay leaf, and serve.
Nutrition: Calories: 585; Total fat: 4g; Protein: 40g; Sodium: 616mg; Fiber: 48g

Moroccan Chickpea Stew

Preparation Time: 15 Minutes Cooking Time: 8 Hours Servings: 4
Ingredients:
- 1 small butternut squash, peeled and chopped into bite-size pieces
- 3 cups Very Easy Vegetable Broth or store-bought
- 1 medium yellow onion, diced

- 1 bell pepper, diced
- 1 (15-ounce) can chickpeas, drained and rinsed
- 1 (14.5-ounce) can tomato sauce
- ¾ cup brown lentils, rinsed

Directions:
- 1½ teaspoons minced garlic (3 cloves)
- 1½ teaspoons ground ginger
- 1½ teaspoons ground turmeric
- 1½ teaspoons ground cumin
- 1 teaspoon ground cinnamon
- ¾ teaspoon smoked paprika
- ½ teaspoon salt
- 1 (8-ounce) package fresh udon noodles
- Freshly ground black pepper

1. Combine the butternut squash, vegetable broth, onion, bell pepper, chickpeas, tomato sauce, brown lentils, garlic, ginger, turmeric, cumin, cinnamon, smoked paprika, and salt in a slow cooker. Mix well.
2. Cover and cook 6 to 8 hours on low or 3 to 4 hours on high. In the last 10 minutes of cooking, add the noodles. Season with pepper, and serve.

Nutrition: Calories: 427; Total fat: 4g; Protein: 26g; Sodium: 1,423mg; Fiber: 24g

Tex-Mex Taco Filling

Preparation Time: 15 Minutes **Cooking Time:** 8 Hours **Servings:** 4

Ingredients:
- 2 cups Very Easy Vegetable Broth or store-bought
- 1 cup green lentils, rinsed
- ½ cup uncooked quinoa, rinsed
- ¼ cup finely diced yellow onion
- 1½ teaspoons minced garlic (3 cloves)
- 2 teaspoons ground cumin
- 1 teaspoon chili powder

Directions:
- ½ teaspoon smoked paprika
- Pinch salt
- Freshly ground black pepper
- Tortillas or taco shells, for serving
- Optional toppings: Nacho Cheese, Guacamole, minced onions, sliced radishes, cilantro, or hot sauce

1. Combine the vegetable broth, lentils, quinoa, onion, garlic, cumin, chili powder, and smoked paprika in a slow cooker. Mix well.
2. Cover and cook on low for 7 to 8 hours.
3. Season with salt and pepper.
4. Serve with tortillas or taco shells and your choice of toppings.

Nutrition: Calories: 283; Total fat: 3g; Protein: 14g; Sodium: 434mg; Fiber: 17g

Ratatouille

Preparation Time: 15 Minutes **Cooking Time:** 6 Hours **Servings:** 4

Ingredients:
- 3 cups peeled diced eggplant
- 1 medium yellow onion, thinly sliced
- 1 green bell pepper, cut into strips
- 1 red bell pepper, cut into strips
- 3 medium zucchinis, sliced
- 2 teaspoons minced garlic (4 cloves)

Directions:
- 1½ (28-ounce) cans plum tomatoes, drained
- 3 tablespoons tomato paste
- 2½ tablespoons olive oil
- Pinch salt, plus more for salting eggplant
- Freshly ground black pepper
- ½ cup chopped fresh basil, for garnish

1. Put the diced eggplant in a colander over the sink, sprinkle with salt, and set aside.
2. Put the onion, bell peppers, zucchini, and garlic in a slow cooker. Pat the eggplant dry and stir it into the slow cooker.
3. Add the tomatoes, tomato paste, and olive oil to the slow cooker and mix thoroughly.
4. Cover and cook on low for 6 hours.
5. Season with salt and pepper. Garnish with the basil and serve.

Nutrition: Calories: 226; Total fat: 10g; Protein: 7g; Sodium: 85mg; Fiber: 7g

Cauliflower Bolognese

Preparation Time: 15 Minutes Cooking Time: 9 Hours Servings: 4
Ingredients:
- ½ head cauliflower, cut into florets
- 1 (8- to 10-ounce) container button mushrooms
- 1 small yellow onion, quartered
- 2 medium carrots, scrubbed and cut into chunks
- 2 cups eggplant chunks
- 2½ teaspoons minced garlic (5 cloves)
- 2 (28-ounce) cans crushed tomatoes
- 2 tablespoons tomato paste

Directions:
- 2 tablespoons cane sugar or agave nectar
- 2 tablespoons balsamic vinegar
- 2 tablespoons nutritional yeast
- 1½ tablespoons dried oregano
- 1½ tablespoons dried basil
- 1½ teaspoons chopped fresh rosemary leaves
- Pinch salt
- Freshly ground black pepper

1. In a food processor, pulse the cauliflower, mushrooms, onion, carrots, eggplant, and garlic until all the vegetables are finely chopped. Transfer to a slow cooker.
2. Add the crushed tomatoes, tomato paste, cane sugar, balsamic vinegar, nutritional yeast, oregano, basil, and rosemary to the slow cooker; mix well.
3. Cover and cook on low for 8 to 9 hours or on high for 4 to 5 hours.
4. Season with salt and pepper, and serve.

Nutrition: Calories: 281; Total fat: 10g; Protein: 17g; Sodium: 855mg; Fiber: 20g

Vegan Cauliflower Rice and Beans

Preparation Time: 5 Minutes Cooking Time: 4 Hours
Servings: 6
Ingredients:
- 24 oz cauliflower rice, frozen
- ½ cup hulled hemp seeds
- 1 cup vegetable stock
- 3 tbsp olive oil
- 2 tbsp garlic powder

- 1 tbsp onion powder

Directions:
- 1 tbsp cumin
- 1 tbsp chili powder
- ½ tbsp cumin
- 1 tbsp chili powder
- ½ tbsp cayenne powder
- 1 tbsp Mexican oregano

1. Add all the ingredients to the slow cooker except oregano, then stir well to mix.
2. Cover the slow cooker and cook on high for 4 hours. The rice should be tender.
3. Garnish as you desire, then serve. Enjoy.

Nutrition: Calories 278, Total Fat 20.2g, Saturated Fat 9g, Total Carbs 4.9g, Net Carbs 2.1g, Protein 19.3g, Sugar: 2g, Fiber: 11.8g

Tomatoes Aubergines

Preparation Time: 15 Minutes Cooking Time: 8 Hours Servings: 6
Ingredients:
- 4 tbsp olive oil - 1 red onion, sliced
- 2 garlic cloves, crushed
- 18 oz aubergines, sliced into 1 cm thick slices
- 11 oz tomatoes, ripe and quartered
- 1 fennel bulb, sliced
- 2 oz tomatoes, sundried
- 1 tbsp coriander seeds

Directions:
For Dressing
- 1 small bunch flat-leaf parsley, roughly chopped
- 1 small bunch basil, roughly chopped
- 1 small bunch chives, roughly chopped
- 2 tbsp olive oil - 1 lemon juice For Topping
- 4 oz feta cheese
- 2 oz flaked almonds, toasted

1. Add 2 tbsp of olive oil to your slow cooker. Add onions and garlic on top.
2. Brush the aubergines with the remaining two tablespoons of oil and place them on garlic.
3. Nestle the ripe tomatoes, fennel bulb slices, and dried tomatoes around the aubergines.
4. Sprinkle coriander seeds and season with salt and pepper. Cover the slow cooker and cook on low for 8 hours.
5. When the time has elapsed, add all the dressing ingredients in a blender and pulse until smooth.
6. Use a slotted spoon to transfer the vegetables to a serving plate. Drizzle dressing, then top with cheese and almonds. Serve and enjoy.

Nutrition: Calories 256, Total Fat 20g, Saturated Fat 4g, Total Carbs 11g, Net Carbs 5g, Protein 8g, Sugar: 9g, Fiber: 6g

Bacon Brussels Sprouts

Preparation Time: 5 Minutes - Cooking Time: 2 Hours Servings: 8
Ingredients:
- 16 oz brussels sprouts, trim ends and half
- 1 tbsp olive oil - 2 tbsp garlic, minced
- ½ tbsp white onion, chopped

Directions:
- 6 slices bacon, chopped
- ½ tbsp salt
- ¼ tbsp black pepper

1. Add water in the slow cooker insert. Arrange brussels sprouts in a steamer basket, then place it on the insert. Cover the slow cooker and cook on high for 2 hours.
2. When the time has elapsed, remove Brussels sprouts from the slow cooker.
3. Add oil in a skillet and sauté garlic and onions for 2 minutes.
4. Add bacon slices to the skillet and cook until crispy. Add brussels sprouts and stir cook for 3 minutes. Serve and enjoy.

Nutrition: Calories 197, Total Fat 13g, Saturated Fat 4g, Total Carbs 12g, Net Carbs 4g, Protein 8g, Sugar: 3g, Fiber: 4g, Sodium: 538mg, Potassium: 526mg

Egg and Broccoli Casserole

Preparation Time: 15 Minutes Cooking Time: 3 Hours
Servings: 6
Ingredients:
- 24 oz cottage cheese
- 3 cups broccoli, chopped when frozen, thawed, and drained
- 2 cup cheddar cheese, shredded
- 6 eggs, beaten lightly

Directions:
- 1/3 cup almond flour
- ¼ cup butter, melted
- 3 tbsp onion, finely chopped
- ½ tbsp salt

1. Add all the ingredients to a mixing bowl and mix well to combine
2. Grease your 3-quart slow cooker and pour the mixture in the slow cooker.
3. Cover the slow cooker and cook on high for 1 hour.
4. Stir, reduce heat to low, and cook for two more hours.
5. Sprinkle with more cheddar cheese if you desire. Serve and enjoy.

Nutrition: Calories 463, Total Fat 30.1g, Saturated Fat 17.5g, Total Carbs 13.1g, Net Carbs 11.7g, Protein 35g, Sugar: 2g, Fiber: 1.4g, Sodium: 1073mg

Delicious Garden Frittata

Preparation Time: 10 Minutes Cooking Time: 3 Hours Servings: 8
Ingredients:
- 1 tbsp olive oil
- ¼ cup scallions, sliced
- 5 oz spinach
- 1 tomato, diced
- ¼ cup mushrooms, sliced

Directions:
- 8 eggs, beaten
- ½ tbsp seasoning salt
- Black pepper to taste
- 5 oz feta cheese, crumbled

1. Heat oil on a skillet and sauté scallions and spinach for 2 minutes.
2. Grease your 6-quart slow cooker with butter, then transfer the sautéed onions and spinach to it.
3. Add tomatoes and mushrooms to the slow cooker.
4. Add eggs and stir well to combine. Season with salt and pepper, then sprinkle cheese.
5. Cover the slow cooker and cook on low for 3 hours.
6. Serve and enjoy.

Nutrition: Calories 171.8, Total Fat 12.2g, Saturated Fat 5.4g, Total Carbs 4.5g, Net Carbs 3.8g, Protein 11g, Sugar: 1.6g, Fiber: 0.7g, Sodium: 329mg, Potassium: 1154mg

Broccoli Cheese Casserole

Preparation Time: 20 Minutes Cooking Time: 4 Hours
Servings: 8
Ingredients:
- 10 ¾ oz cream of mushroom soup, condensed
- 1 cup mayonnaise
- 1 tbsp garlic powder
- 1 egg, beaten

Directions:
1. Grease your 4-quart slow cooker insert.
- ½ yellow onion, finely chopped
- Salt and pepper
- 30 oz broccoli, frozen chopped
- 8 oz + 2 oz cheddar cheese, shredded
- 2 pinches paprika

2. Mix cream of mushroom soup, mayonnaise, garlic powder, eggs, onion, salt, and pepper in a mixing bowl.
3. Break up broccoli in a separate mixing bowl, then pour the mayonnaise mixture over the broccoli. Mix well.
4. Add 8 oz cheese and mix again, then transfer the mixture to your slow cooker. Spread the mixture evenly in the slow cooker.
5. Cover the slow cooker and cook on high for 4 hours.
6. When the time has elapsed, sprinkle the remaining cheese, then cover and cook for 15 more minutes.
7. Serve and enjoy.

Nutrition: Calories 300, Total Fat 21.2g, Saturated Fat 7.9g, Total Carbs 16.1g, Net Carbs 13.3g, Protein 11.3g, Sugar: 4.3g, Fiber: 2.9g, Sodium: 623mg, Potassium: 393mg

Chicken Butter Mushrooms

Preparation Time: 5 Minutes Cooking Time: 4 Hours
Servings: 2
Ingredients:
- 1 lb. mushrooms, cleaned and sliced
- ½ cup butter
- 1 tbsp Marjoram
- 1 tbsp chives, minced

Directions:
- Salt and pepper to taste
- ½ cup chicken or vegetable broth
- ¼ cup dry white wine

1. Place the mushroom in the slow cooker and add butter on top.
2. Mix all other ingredients in a mixing bowl and pour on top of the mushrooms and butter.
3. Cover the slow cooker and cook on low for 4 hours. The mushrooms should be tender.
4. Serve and enjoy.

Nutrition: Calories 497, Total Fat 47.2g, Saturated Fat 29.4g, Total Carbs 9.1g, Net Carbs 6.5g, Protein 8.9g, Sugar: 4.2g, Fiber: 2.6g, Sodium: 531mg

Brunch Florentine

Preparation Time: 12 Minutes Cooking Time: 2 Hours Servings: 5
Ingredients:
- Cooking spray
- 1 ½ cup cheddar cheese, grated and divided
- 9 oz frozen spinach, thawed and drained
- 1 cup button mushrooms, freshly sliced
- ½ cup green onions, sliced thinly

Directions:
1. Spray your slow cooker lightly with cooking spray.
- 6 eggs
- ½ cup heavy cream
- 1 ½ cup milk
- 1 tbsp garlic powder
- 1 tbsp salt
- 1 tbsp black pepper, freshly ground

2. Scatter half cheddar cheese at the bottom of the slow cooker, then layer spinach, mushrooms, and onions on the cheese.
3. Whisk together eggs, heavy cream, milk, garlic powder, salt, and black pepper in a mixing bowl.
4. Pour the egg mixture over the layered ingredients in the slow cooker.
5. Sprinkle the remaining cheese, then cover the slow cooker and cook on high for 2 hours.
6. Serve and enjoy.

Nutrition: Calories 245, Total Fat 15.4g, Saturated Fat 8.2g, Total Carbs 9.9g, Net Carbs 8.4g, Protein 16.8g, Sugar: 4.7g, Fiber: 1.5g, Sodium: 724mg, Potassium: 136mg

Fire Roasted Tomato Soup

Preparation Time: 15 Minutes **Cooking Time:** 7 Hours
Servings: 10
Ingredients:
- 2 tbsp coconut oil
- 2 yellow onion, thinly sliced
- 1 tbsp sea salt
- 1 ½ tbsp curry powder
- 1 tbsp coriander, ground

Directions:
- 1 tbsp cumin
- ¼ tbsp red pepper flakes
- 56 oz whole tomatoes, fire-roasted
- 5 cups of water
- 14 oz can coconut milk

1. Melt oil on a skillet, then sauté onions until tender. Make sure they do not burn.
2. Add seasonings and spices and cook for one more minute.
3. Transfer the sautéed onion mixture to the slow cooker. Add tomatoes and water to the slow cooker.
4. Cover the slow cooker and cook on low for 6 hours.
5. When the time has elapsed, use an immersion blender to blend the soup until smooth.
6. Add coconut milk and cook for one more hour. Serve and enjoy.

Nutrition: Calories 192, Total Fat 15.3g, Saturated Fat 13.1g, Total Carbs 10.9g, Net Carbs 7.4g, Protein 2.7g, Sugar: 6.4g, Fiber: 3.5g, Sodium: 202mg

Vegetable Cheese Frittata

Preparation Time: 5 Minutes **Cooking Time:** 2 Hours
Servings: 4
Ingredients:
- 1 tbsp ghee
- 4 oz sliced mushrooms
- ¼ tbsp fresh chopped spinach
- ¼ cup sliced tomatoes
- 2 sliced green onions

Directions:
- 6 eggs

- 2 tbsp Italian seasoning
- ½ cup cheese
- 1 tbsp parmesan cheese

1. Prepare your slow cooker by generously spraying with cooking spray.
2. Meanwhile, melt ghee in a medium frying pan.
3. Add vegetables, then sauté for a few minutes until soft.
4. Whisk together eggs, seasonings, and cheeses in a bowl.
5. Pour the mixture into your slow cooker and cover.
6. Cook for about 3-4 hours on low or 1-2 hours on high.
7. Serve and enjoy.

Nutrition: Calories: 13.3g, Saturated fat: 5.9g, Total carbs: 3.2g, Net carbs: 2.3g, Protein: 14.3g, Sugars: 1.4g, Fiber: 0.9g, Sodium: 1018mg, Potassium: 743mg

Beefy Vegetable Soup

Preparation Time: 15 Minutes Cooking Time: 6 Hours Servings: 10
Ingredients:
- 2 lbs. drained and browned beef, ground
- 2 cups beef broth
- 24½ oz marinara sauce
- 1 chopped zucchini, medium
- 1 chopped yellow squash, medium
- ¼ chopped celery ribs

Directions:
- 1 cup chopped radishes
- 2 cups chopped cabbage
- 2 tbsp garlic, minced
- Pepper and salt to taste
- *For garnish:* shredded cheese

1. Place all the ingredients into a slow cooker, 6-8 quart, except shredded cheese.
2. Stir and cover your slow cooker.
3. Cook for about 6-8 hours on low or 4-5 hours on high until veggies become tender.
4. Serve and enjoy.

Nutrition: Calories: 269, Total fat: 19g, Saturated fat: 7g, Total carbs: 8g, Net carbs: 6g, Protein: 18g, Sugars: 5g, Fiber: 2g, Sodium: 626mg, Potassium: 708mg

Zucchini Lasagna

Preparation Time: 15 Minutes Cooking Time: 3 Hours Servings: 6
Ingredients:
- 1½ lbs. zucchini, ends cut
- 1-2 tbsp salt
- 24 oz marinara sauce
- 15 oz ricotta cheese

Directions:
- 8 oz shredded provolone
- 8 oz shredded parmesan cheese
- *For garnish: fresh basil*

1. Slice the zucchini lengthwise to ¼" strips, then splash with 1 tbsp salt. Let sit for about 20-30 minutes.
2. Cover using a paper towel and squeeze out water, patting them dry. Add salt and repeat if you still have more water.
3. Place ½ cup marinara sauce to your slow cooker bottom, then place a layer of 1/3 noodles, ricotta cheese, provolone, and more sauce. Repeat the process to have three layers.
4. Top with cheese, parmesan cheese, and remaining sauce.

5. Cover your slow cooker and cook for about 4-6 hours on low or 2-3 hours on high or until noodles become tender.
6. Uncover and let sit for 15-20 minutes.
7. Slice and garnish with basil.
8. Serve and enjoy.

Nutrition: Calories: 433, Total Fat: 29g, Saturated fat: 18g, Total Carbs: 13g, Net carbs: 11g, Protein: 30g, Sugars: 8g, Fiber: 2g, Sodium: 1682mg, Potassium: 826mg

Pumpkin and Coconut Soup

Preparation Time: 10 Minutes Cooking Time: 4 Hours
Servings: 6
Ingredients:
- 1 diced onion, medium
- 1 tbsp crushed ginger
- 1 tbsp crushed garlic
- 4 tbsp butter

Directions:
- 2 lbs. pumpkin chunks
- 2 cups vegetable stock
- 1½ cup coconut cream
- Pepper and salt to taste

1. Place all ingredients in your slow cooker. Mix and cover.
2. Cook for about 6-8 hours on low or 4-6 hours on high.
3. Use an immersion blender to puree the soup until smooth.
4. Garnish using coconut cream.
5. Serve warm and enjoy.

Nutrition: Calories: 234, Total Fat: 21.7g, Saturated fat: 11.4g, Total carbs: 11.4g, Net carbs: 9.9g, Protein: 2.3g, Sugars: 6.4g, Fiber: 1.5g, Sodium: 359mg, Potassium: 117mg

Crustless Spinach Quiche

Preparation Time: 15 Minutes Cooking Time: 3 Hours Servings: 6
Ingredients:
- Non-stick cooking spray
- 4 eggs
- ½ tbsp salt
- Ground pepper
- 1 cup half and half
- 2 cups ham, cubed,

Directions:
1. Greece your slow cooker with cooking spray
- 4 shredded Mexican cheese, ½ cup Sargento
- ½ cup Sargento sharp shredded cheddar cheese
- 3 cups spinach, washed,

2. Beat your eggs in a medium bowl, add in salt, pepper, half and half, ham, cheese, and spinach, then stir. Pour your mixture into the slow cooker and cover.
3. Cook for 3 hours on high or 5 hours on low.
4. Slice and serve the quiche.

Nutrition: Calories 216, Total Fat 14.1g, Saturated Fat 6.6g, Total Carbs 4.6g, Net Carbs 3.7g, Protein 15.9g, Sugar 0.4g, Fiber 0.9g, Sodium 1313, Potassium 305mg.

Vegetarian Tikka Masala

Preparation Time: 10 Minutes Cooking Time: 8 Hours Servings: 6

Ingredients:
- 3 cups cubed rutabagas
- 4 cups cauliflower florets
- 2 cucumbers peeled and sliced into 1" diagonal pieces
- 4 minced garlic cloves
- ½ diced yellow onions
- 3 cups vegetable broth, lower-sodium
- 15 oz crushed tomatoes
- 3 tbsp tomato paste

Directions:
- 2 tbsp garam masala
- ¾ tbsp ground ginger
- 1 tbsp paprika
- 1 tbsp kosher salt
- 1 cup of canned coconut milk
- ¾ cup snow peas, frozen and thawed
- Cooked cauliflower rice
- Fresh cilantro for garnish

1. Combine all ingredients in your slow cooker except peas, coconut milk, cilantro, and rice.
2. Cook while covered until vegetables are tender for about 8-9 hours on low or 4-5 hours on high.
3. Turn off your slow cooker, then stir in coconut milk and peas.
4. Wait for 5 minutes when covered before serving.
5. Garnish with cilantro and serve with rice.

Nutrition: Calories 268, Total Fat 21.2g, Saturated Fat 13.7g, Total Carbs 14.5g, Net Carbs 8.9g, Protein 4.7g, Sugar 5.3g, Fiber 5.6g, Sodium 298mg, Potassium 716mg.

CHAPTER 10: SOUPS

Creamy Chicken Soup

Preparation Time: 5 Minutes Cooking Time: 8 Hours
Servings: 4
Ingredients:
- 3 cooked + shredded chicken breasts
- 4 cups chicken stock
- 1 cup heavy cream
- 2 chopped carrots - 2 chopped celery stalks

Directions:
- 1 diced sweet onion
- 2 minced garlic cloves
- 1 teaspoon dried thyme
- Salt and pepper to taste

1. Put all the ingredients (except cream) into your slow cooker.
2. Cook on low for 8 hours. When there are thirty minutes left to go, add cream.
3. When time is up, taste and season more with salt and pepper if needed. Serve hot!

Nutrition: Total calories: 123, Protein: 16, Carbs: 10, Fat: 3, Fiber: 1

Mexican Chicken Soup

Preparation Time: 10 Minutes Cooking Time: 2 Hours Servings: 4
Ingredients:
- 32-ounces chicken broth
- One 28-ounce can of tomatoes
- 2 chopped cooked chicken breasts
- 2 seeded and diced jalapeno peppers
- 1 cup of water - 1 chopped red onion
- 4 minced garlic cloves

Directions:
- 2 tablespoons no-sugar tomato paste
- 1 handful of chopped parsley
- 1 teaspoon cumin
- ½ teaspoon chili powder
- Drizzle of olive oil
- Salt and pepper to taste

1. Pour oil into a skillet and heat. When hot, add ¼ cup broth, jalapenos, onion, garlic, salt, and pepper.
2. When the onions and peppers are soft, pour into the slow cooker.
3. Pour in the rest of the ingredients except parsley.
4. Close the lid. Cook on low for 2 hours. Chicken should be 165-degrees and very tender.
5. Shred chicken and serve!

Nutrition: Total calories: 135, Protein: 13, Carbs: 20, Fat: 3, Fiber: 2.5

Thai-Inspired Chicken Soup

Preparation Time: 10 Minutes Cooking Time: 8 Hours
Servings: 8 to 10
Ingredients:
- 1 whole organic chicken
- One 14-ounce can of full-fat coconut milk
- 4-inch thumb of chopped ginger
- 1 chopped lemongrass stalk

Directions:
- Enough vegetable broth to cover the chicken
- Splash of Red Boat fish sauce
- Salt to taste

1. Put the whole chicken, ginger, and lemongrass in your slow cooker.
2. Pour in coconut milk and enough vegetable broth to cover the chicken.
3. Close the lid.
4. Cook on low for 8-10 hours.
5. When time is up, remove the chicken, and pull all the meat off the bones.
6. Return meat to the soup.
7. Taste and season with salt and fish sauce as needed.
8. Serve!

Nutrition: Total calories: 330, Protein: 22, Carbs: 2, Fat: 26, Fiber: 0

Spicy Pepper Chicken Soup

Preparation Time: 5 Minutes Cooking Time: 6 to 8 Hours
Servings: 6
Ingredients:
- 3 chopped raw chicken breasts
- 8-ounces chicken stock
- 2 seeded and chopped jalapeno peppers
- 1 chopped poblano chili pepper
- ½ cup chopped green onions
- 3 minced garlic cloves

Directions:
- 5 teaspoons 100% natural peanut butter
- 4 teaspoons coconut aminos
- 4 teaspoons lime juice
- ½ tablespoon+ crushed red pepper flakes
- 1 teaspoon ground ginger
- Salt and pepper to taste

1. The night before you plan on making the soup, put all the ingredients (minus green onions) in your slow cooker.
2. Marinate in the fridge overnight.
3. When you're ready to cook, remove the slow cooker and wait 20 minutes before turning it on.
4. Turn to low and cook for 6-8 hours.
5. Taste and add more red pepper flakes if you want more heat.
6. Garnish with chopped green onions and serve!

Nutrition: Total calories: 102, Protein: 13, Carbs: 4, Fat: 4, Fiber: 0

Turkey + Herbs Soup

Preparation Time: 5 Minutes Cooking Time: 2 Hours
Servings: 4
Ingredients:
- 4 cups turkey/chicken stock
- 3 cups cooked turkey meat
- 3 cups chopped fresh spinach
- 1 cup chopped onion
- 2 fresh rosemary sprigs

Directions:
1. Melt the butter in a skillet and add onions.
2. Cook until soft.

- ½ tablespoon grass-fed butter
- 1 teaspoon garlic powder
- ½ teaspoon dried parsley
- ½ teaspoon dried thyme
- Salt and pepper to taste

3. Add to your slow cooker with the rest of the ingredients (except spinach).
4. Close the lid.
5. Cook for 2 hours on low. Since there isn't anything raw in the recipe, you're just simmering the flavors together.
6. A few minutes before serving, stir in the spinach, and let the soup's heat wilt the greens.
7. Taste and season with more salt and pepper if needed. Enjoy!

Nutrition: Total calories: 331, Protein: 19, Carbs: 6, Fat: 26, Fiber: 0

Beefy Chili

Preparation Time: 10 Minutes Cooking Time: 6 Hours Servings: 6
Ingredients:
- 21-ounces ground beef
- 21-ounces stew beef
- One 8-ounce can have diced tomatoes
- 1 cup beef stock
- 2 chopped sweet onions

Directions:
1. Heat olive oil in a skillet.
2. When hot, add garlic and onions.
3. Cook until softened.
4. Put into your slow cooker.
5. Add the rest of the ingredients.
6. Close the lid.
7. Cook on low for 4-6 hours.
- 4 minced garlic cloves
- 1 tablespoon red chili flakes
- Splash of extra virgin olive oil
- Salt and pepper to taste

8. Ground beef should be 160-degrees, while steak can be 145-degrees.
9. Serve hot!

Nutrition: Total calories: 325, Protein: 40, Carbs: 6, Fat: 16, Fiber: 0

Shredded Pork Chili

Preparation Time: 15 Minutes Cooking Time: 8 to 10 Hours
Servings: 6 to 8
Ingredients:
- 2 pounds pork roast
- Two 14-ounce cans of diced tomatoes
- One 14-ounce can of no-sugar tomato sauce
- 2 chopped yellow bell peppers
- 2 chopped sweet onions
- 3 wholes + peeled garlic cloves

Directions:
1. Trim any excess fat from the pork.
2. Put in your slow cooker.
- 1 seeded and chopped jalapeno pepper
- ½ cup Frank's Original hot sauce

- 2 tablespoons paprika
- 2 tablespoons onion powder
- 1 tablespoon cumin
- Salt and pepper to taste

3. Cut three slashes into the roast (one on top, two on the sides) and stick in the whole garlic cloves.
4. Season well with the spices.
5. Pour in hot sauce, onion, jalapeno, tomato sauce, tomatoes, and bell peppers over the roast.
6. Close the lid. Cook on low for 8-10 hours.
7. Pork should be at least 145-degrees at its thickest part.
8. Shred up the pork and stir. Taste and add more salt if needed.
9. If you want it spicier, add more hot sauce.
10. Serve hot!

Nutrition: Total calories: 408, Protein: 33, Carbs: 21, Fat: 22, Fiber: 2.8

Beef Minestrone

Preparation Time: 15 Minutes Cooking Time: 5 to 8 Hours
Servings: 4
Ingredients:
- 1-pound grass-fed ground beef
- 3 cups hot water
- 28-ounces diced tomatoes
- 2 diced zucchinis - 1 diced onion
- 1 diced celery stalk- 1 diced carrot

Directions:
- ½ cup vegetable broth
- 3 minced garlic cloves
- ½ teaspoon dried oregano
- ½ teaspoon onion powder

1. Heat a skillet. Add your ground beef and cook until just browned. While the beef is browning, heat 3 cups of water in a separate pot until boiling.
2. Pour beef and water into the slow cooker.
3. Add in the rest of the ingredients. Close the lid. Cook on low for 5-8 hours.
4. Taste and season. Serve!

Nutrition: Total calories: 275, Protein: 26, Carbs: 12, Fat: 15, Fiber: 3.5

Cream of Broccoli-Cauliflower Soup

Preparation Time: 10 Minutes Cooking Time: 3 Hours Servings: 4
Ingredients:
- 8 cups of broccoli florets
- 4 cups cauliflower florets
- 3 cups chicken stock
- 1cupfull-fatcoconutmilk(room temperature)

Directions:
1. Heat olive oil in a skillet and add onion and garlic.
- 1 chopped celery stalk - 1 chopped onion
- 1 tablespoon extra-virgin olive oil
- 2 minced garlic cloves
- ½ teaspoon onion powder
- Salt and pepper to taste

2. Cook for 3 minutes until the onion has softened a bit.
3. Add all the ingredients (except coconut milk) into your slow cooker.
4. Close the lid. Cook on low for 3 hours.

5. When time is up, puree using an immersion blender. If you don't have an immersion blender, carefully blend the soup in batches in a regular blender.
6. Return smooth soup to a slow cooker. Stir in room-temperature coconut milk.
7. Taste and season more if necessary!
Nutrition: Total calories: 283, Protein: 29, Carbs: 23, Fat: 14, Fiber: 6

Cheesy Cauliflower Chowder w/ Bacon

Preparation Time: 10 Minutes Cooking Time: 3 to 4 Hours
Servings: 8
Ingredients:
- 4 cups shredded cauliflower
- 2 ½ cups cheddar cheese
- 2 cups full-fat coconut milk
- 2 cups chicken stock- 8 slices bacon
- 2 minced garlic cloves

Directions:
- 1 chopped celery stalk
- 1 tablespoon coconut flour
- Dash of hot sauce
- ½ teaspoon onion powder
- Salt and pepper to taste

1. Cook bacon in a skillet until crisp. Wrap in a paper towel for now. In a small bowl, mix coconut flour into your chicken stock until smooth.
2. Put this mixture and all the ingredients (minus coconut milk, cheese, and bacon) into your slow cooker. Close the lid.
3. Cook for 3-4 hours on low.
4. When time is up, puree soup with an immersion blender or in batches with a regular blender.
5. Stir in room-temperature coconut milk.
6. Top with cheese and crumbled bacon!
Nutrition: Total calories: 351, Protein: 17, Carbs: 6, Fat: 27, Fiber: 1.6

Ham + Pumpkin Soup

Preparation Time: 5 Minutes Cooking Time: 6 Hours
Servings: 8 to 10
Ingredients:
- 2 pounds ham hock
- 2 pounds' worth of small diced pumpkins
- Enough boiling water to cover

Directions:
1. Put ham hock and pumpkin in your slow cooker.
2. Cover with boiling water.
3. Close the lid.
4. Cook on low for 6-10 hours.
- Salt and pepper to taste
- ½ teaspoon dried sage
- Pinch of nutmeg
5. When that time is up, remove the hock and pull the meat away from the bones.
6. Put the meat back in your cooker.
7. With an immersion blender, carefully puree until smooth, or use a regular blender and puree in batches.
8. Season well with salt, pepper, dried sage, and a pinch of nutmeg.
9. Serve!
Nutrition: Total calories: 347, Protein: 25, Carbs: 3, Fat: 24, Fiber: 0

Cream of Zucchini Soup

Preparation Time: 5 Minutes Cooking Time: 2 Hours
Servings: 4
Ingredients:
- 3 cups vegetable stock
- 2 pounds chopped zucchini
- 2 minced garlic cloves
- ¾ cup chopped onion

Directions:
1. Heat olive oil in a skillet.
- ¼ cup basil leaves
- 1 tablespoon extra-virgin olive oil
- Salt and pepper to taste

2. When hot, cook garlic and onion for about 5 minutes.
3. Pour into your slow cooker with the rest of the ingredients.
4. Close the lid.
5. Cook on low for 2 hours.
6. When time is up, puree the soup with an immersion blender or batches in a regular blender.
7. Taste and season more if needed!

Nutrition: Total Calories: 96, Protein: 7, Carbs: 11, Fat: 5, Fiber: 2.3

Tomato Soup

Preparation Time: 5 Minutes Cooking Time: 4 Hours
Servings: 4
Ingredients:
- One 28-ounce can of crushed tomatoes
- 1 cup vegetable broth
- ½ cup heavy cream
- 2 tablespoons chopped parsley

Directions:
- ½ teaspoon onion powder
- ½ teaspoon garlic powder
- Salt and pepper to taste

1. Put all the ingredients (except cream) in the slow cooker.
2. Cook on low for 4 hours.
3. When time is up, blend the soup with an immersion blender or batches with a regular blender.
4. Stir in the cream.
5. Taste and season with more salt and pepper if necessary.

Nutrition: Total Calories: 165, Protein: 3, Carbs: 15, Fat: 13, Fiber: 3.7

Vegetable Korma (Stew)

Preparation Time: 5 Minutes Cooking Time: 8 Hours
Servings: 4
Ingredients:
- 1 head's worth of cauliflower florets
- ¾ of a 10-ounce can of full-fat coconut milk
- 2 cups chopped green beans
- ½ chopped onion

Directions:
1. Add vegetables into your slow cooker.
2. Mix coconut milk with seasonings.
3. Pour into the slow cooker.

4. Sprinkle over coconut flour and mix until blended.
5. Close the lid.
6. Cook on low for 8 hours.
7. Taste and season more if necessary.
8. Serve!
- 2 minced garlic cloves
- 2 tablespoons curry powder
- 2 tablespoons coconut flour
- 1 teaspoon garam masala
- Salt and pepper to taste

Nutrition: Total Calories: 206, Protein: 5, Carbs: 18, Fat: 14, Fiber: 9.5

CHAPTER 11: DESSERTS

Raspberry Yogurt

Preparation Time: 20 Minutes Cooking Time: 12 Hours Servings: 3
Ingredients:
- 8 cups whole milk, pasteurized
- ½ cup natural, plain yogurt

Directions:
- ½ cup raspberries
- Thick bath towel

1. Pour milk in the slow cooker and cook, covered on LOW for about 2 hours.
2. Allow it to sit for about 3 hours. Scoop out 2 cups of the warm milk into a bowl.
3. Add yogurt and return to the one-pot slow cooker, stirring well.
4. Cover the lid and wrap it with a heavy bath towel.
5. Let it sit for about 7 hours and transfer to an immersion blender along with the raspberries.
6. Transfer to a plastic container in the refrigerator and serve after set.

Nutrition: Calories: 421, Fat: 21g, Carbohydrates: 32g

Banana Bread

Preparation Time: 30 Minutes Cooking Time: 3 Hours Servings: 5
Ingredients:
- 1 teaspoon baking soda
- ½ cup pecans, chopped and lightly toasted
- 2 cups flour
- 1 teaspoon salt
- ½ cup butter softened

Directions:
- 1 cup of sugar
- 4 small bananas, ripe and mashed
- 1 teaspoon vanilla
- 2 eggs
- 2 tablespoons plus 2 teaspoons milk

1. Mix baking soda, flour, and salt in a bowl and add nuts.
2. Mix butter, eggs, sugar, vanilla, milk, and bananas in another bowl.
3. Add the flour mixture gradually and mix well.
4. Place insert into the slow cooker and add batter.
5. Cover and cook on HIGH for about 3 hours.

Nutrition: Calories: 618, Fat: 23.1g, Carbohydrates: 97.7g

Rice Pudding with Mixed Berries

Preparation Time: 10 Minutes Cooking Time: 7 Hours and 30 Minutes Servings: 6
Ingredients:
- 1 package (4 ounces) dried blueberries
- 1½ cups water
- 1 cup heavy cream
- 1 package (6 ounces) dried cranberries
- 1 can (12 ounces) evaporated milk

Directions:
- 8 ounces frozen orange juice concentrate
- ¾ cup of sugar
- A dash of salt

- 1 cup short-grain Arborio rice
- ¼ teaspoon ground cinnamon

1. Grease the one pot of the slow cooker with nonstick cooking spray.
2. Mix all the ingredients and pour into the slow cooker.
3. Cover and cook on LOW for about 5 hours.
4. Stir the mixture after 2 hours 30 minutes and dish out after complete time.

Nutrition: Calories: 349, Fat: 12.3g, Carbohydrates: 56.6g

Banana Raisin Bread Pudding

Preparation Time: 15 Minutes Cooking Time: 5 Hours
Servings: 8
Ingredients:
- 2 tablespoons ground cinnamon
- 5 eggs, beaten
- ¾ cup packed brown sugar
- 3½ cups milk
- 6 cups plain breadcrumbs

Directions:
- 1 tablespoon butter, melted
- 2 teaspoons vanilla
- ½ teaspoon salt
- ½ cup raisins
- 1 mashed banana

1. Mix all ingredients until the mixture is smooth like thick oatmeal.
2. Place mixture in a greased slow cooker and cover the lid.
3. Cook on high for about 5 hours and dish out.

Nutrition: Calories: 525, Fat: 10.8g, Carbohydrates: 89.1g

Chocolate Peanut Butter Cups

Preparation Time: 15 Minutes Cooking Time: 5 Hours
Servings: 6
Ingredients:
- ¼ cup heavy cream - ½ cup of sugar
- 1 cup butter

Directions:
- ¼ cup peanut butter, separated
- 2 ounces of milk chocolate

1. Melt the butter and peanut butter, and add milk chocolate, heavy cream, and sugar.
2. Stir thoroughly and put the mixture in a baking mold. Put the baking mold in the slow cooker and cover the lid. Cook on LOW for about 5 hours and dish out to serve hot.

Nutrition: Calories: 465, Fat: 40.7g, Carbohydrates: 24.6g

Flourless Chocolate Brownies

Preparation Time: 20 Minutes Cooking Time: 5 Hours
Servings: 6
Ingredients:
- ¼ cup of sugar - 1 teaspoon vanilla extract
- ½ cup sugar-free chocolate chips

Directions:
- ½ cup butter
- 3 eggs

1. Put eggs, sugar, and vanilla extract in the blender and blend until frothy.

2. Melt butter and chocolate in a bowl and combine with the egg mixture.
3. Pour it into the baking mold and place the mold in the slow cooker. Cover and cook on LOW for about 5 hours. Dish out to serve hot.
Nutrition: Calories: 21g, Fat: 18.1g, Carbohydrates: 10.1g

Crème Brulee

Preparation Time: 15 Minutes Cooking Time: 4 Hours Servings: 4
Ingredients:
- 3 egg yolks - ½ tablespoon vanilla extract
- ¼ cup of sugar - 1 cup heavy cream

Directions:
- 1 pinch salt

1. Put all the ingredients except sugar in a bowl and beat until well combined.
2. Divide the mixture in the ramekins evenly and transfer to the slow cooker.
3. Cover and cook on LOW for about 4 hours. Cover the ramekins with a plastic wrap and refrigerate to chill before serving.
Nutrition: Calories: 195, Fat: 14.5g, Carbohydrates: 14g

Chocolate Cheese Cake

Preparation Time: 15 Minutes Cooking Time: 6 Hours Servings: 4
Ingredients:
- 2 cups cream cheese, softened
- 2 eggs
- ½ cup of sugar

Directions:
- 1 teaspoon pure vanilla extract
- 2 tablespoons cocoa powder

1. Put eggs and cream cheese in a blender and blend until smooth.
2. Add remaining ingredients and pulse until well combined.
3. Transfer the mixture into 2 (8-ounce) mason jars evenly.
4. Put the mason jars in the slow cooker.
5. Set the slow cooker on low and cook for about 6 hours.
6. Refrigerate to chill for at least 6 hours before serving.
Nutrition: Calories: 539, Fat: 43g, Carbohydrates: 29.9g

Peanut Butter Pudding

Preparation Time: 15 Minutes Cooking Time: 6 Hours Servings: 4
Ingredients:
- ½ cup of sugar
- 2 cups cashew milk
- ½ cup of cold water

Directions:
- 2 teaspoons gelatin
- ¼ cup natural peanut butter

1. Put cashew milk, peanut butter, and sugar in the slow cooker and stir well.
2. Cover and cook on LOW for about 2 hours.
3. Mix the gelatin in cold water and transfer it to the slow cooker.
4. Stir for 5 minutes and allow the pudding to sit for 1 hour.
5. Pour into ramekins and refrigerate for 3 hours.
Nutrition: Calories: 270, Fat: 11g, Carbohydrates: 36.5g

Coconut Yogurt

Preparation Time: 5 Minutes Cooking Time: 12 Hours
Servings: 6
Ingredients:
- 1 small container of yogurt
- 3 cups of coconut milk
- 3 tablespoons sugar

Directions:
- 1 tablespoon coconut, shredded
- 3 teaspoons gelatin

1. Preheat the slow cooker on HIGH and add coconut milk.
2. Cover and cook on LOW for about 2 hours.
3. Turn off the heat and add gelatin, yogurt, shredded coconut, and sugar.
4. Wrap the entire slow cooker in beach towels and allow it to sit for 10 hours while the yogurt cultures.

Nutrition: Calories: 332, Fat: 28.9g, Carbohydrates: 16g

Delicious Pumpkin Custard

Preparation Time: 10 Minutes Cooking Time: 2 Hours and 30 Minutes Servings: 6
Ingredients:
- 4 large eggs
- 4 Tbsp coconut oil, melted
- 1 tsp pumpkin pie spice
- 1/2 cup almond flour

Directions:
1. Spray the inside of a slow cooker with cooking spray.
- 1 tsp vanilla
- 1 cup pumpkin purée
- 1/2 cup erythritol
- Pinch of salt
2. Add eggs to a large mixing bowl and blend until smooth using a hand mixer. Slowly beat in the sweetener.
3. Add vanilla and pumpkin purée to the egg mixture and blend well.
4. Add almond flour, pumpkin pie spice, salt, and coconut oil and blend until well combined.
5. Pour mixture into the slow cooker.
6. Place a paper towel on the slow cooker and cover.
7. Cook on low for 2 hours 30 minutes.
8. Cut into servings, serve and enjoy.

Nutrition: Calories 196, Fat 17.2 g, Carbohydrates 5.8 g

Lemon Blueberry Cake

Preparation Time: 10 Minutes Cooking Time: 3 Hours Servings: 12
Ingredients:
- 6 eggs, separated
- ½ cup fresh blueberries
- 2 cups heavy cream
- 1/2 cup Swerve

Directions:
- 1/3 cup fresh lemon juice
- 1 tsp lemon zest
- 1/2 cup coconut flour
- 1/2 tsp salt

1. Add egg whites to a large mixing bowl and beat until stiff peaks form. Set aside.
2. In another bowl, whisk egg yolks with heavy cream, Swerve, lemon juice, lemon zest, coconut flour, and salt. Slowly fold the egg whites into the egg yolk mixture until well combined.

3. Spray the inside of a slow cooker with cooking spray. Pour prepared batter into the slow cooker.
4. Sprinkle blueberries on top of batter. Cover and cook on low for 3 hours.
5. Allow to cool completely, cut, and serve.
Nutrition: Calories 108, Fat 9.7 g, Carbohydrates 2.2 g

Tasty Lemon Cake

Preparation Time: 10 Minutes Cooking Time: 3 Hours Servings: 8
Ingredients:
- 2 eggs
- Zest of 1 lemon
- 1 Tbsp lemon juice
- 1/2 cup whipping cream
- 1/2 cup butter, melted
- 2 tsp baking powder
- 6 Tbsp Swerve
- 1/2 cup coconut flour

Directions:
- 1 1/2 cups almond flour For topping:
- 2 Tbsp fresh lemon juice
- 2 Tbsp butter, melted
- 1/2 cup hot water
- 3 Tbsp Swerve

1. In a mixing bowl, mix almond flour, baking powder, Swerve, and coconut flour.
2. In a large bowl, whisk together eggs, lemon zest, one tablespoon lemon juice, butter, and whipping cream. Add almond flour mixture to the egg mixture and stir until well combined.
3. Spray the inside of a slow cooker with cooking spray. Pour batter into the slow cooker and spread well. In a bowl, combine all topping ingredients and pour over the cake batter. Cover and cook on high for 3 hours.
4. Serve warm cut into squares, and enjoy.
Nutrition: Calories 294, Fat 28.5 g, Carbohydrates 7.4 g

Chocolate Cake

Preparation Time: 10 Minutes Cooking Time: 2 Hours and 30 Minutes Servings: 10
Ingredients:
- 3 large eggs
- 1/2 tsp vanilla
- 2/3 cup unsweetened almond milk
- 6 Tbsp butter, melted
- 1 1/2 tsp baking powder

Directions:
1. Spray a slow cooker inside with cooking spray.
- 3 Tbsp whey protein powder
- 1/2 cup unsweetened cocoa powder
- 1/2 cup Swerve
- 1 cup almond flour
- Pinch of salt

2. In a mixing bowl, whisk together almond flour, baking powder, protein powder, cocoa powder, Swerve, and salt.
3. Stir in eggs, vanilla, almond milk, and butter until well combined.
4. Pour batter into the slow cooker. Cover and cook on low for 2 1/2 hours.
5. Serve warm, cut into squares, and enjoy.
Nutrition: Calories 176, Fat 15 g, Carbohydrates 6.3 g

Coconut Raspberry Cake

Preparation Time: 10 Minutes Cooking Time: 3 Hours Servings: 10
Ingredients:
- 4 large eggs
- 1 cup raspberries
- 1 tsp vanilla
- 3/4 cup unsweetened coconut milk
- 1/2 cup coconut oil, melted
- 2 tsp baking soda

Directions:
- 1/4 cup powdered egg whites
- 3/4 cup Swerve
- 1 cup unsweetened shredded coconut
- 2 cups almond flour
- Pinch of salt

1. Spray a slow cooker inside with cooking spray. In a mixing bowl, whisk together almond flour, baking soda, powdered egg whites, Swerve, shredded coconut, and salt.
2. Stir in eggs, vanilla, coconut milk, and coconut oil until well combined.
3. Add raspberries and fold well. Pour batter into the slow cooker and spread well.
4. Cover and cook on low for 3 hours.
5. Slice, serve, and enjoy.

Nutrition: Calories 382, Fat 34.9 g, Carbohydrates 10.1 g

APPENDIX : RECIPES INDEX

A

African Sweet Potato Stew 80
Almond Granola 40
Aloo Gobi 77
Amazing Pulled Pork 23
Aromatic Jalapeno Wings 57
Asparagus Smoked Salmon 19

B

Bacon & Cheese Frittata 18
Bacon Brussels Sprouts 84
Bacon-Wrapped Cauliflower 34
Baked Beans 77
Balsamic Beef 65
Balsamic Lamb Chops 65
Banana Bread 98
Banana Raisin Bread Pudding 99
Barbacoa Lamb 69
Barbeque Chicken Wings 58
BBQ Beef Burritos 71
Beef & Broccoli 73
Beef and Scallions Bowl 64
Beef and Zucchini Wraps 38
Beef Bourguignon with Carrot Noodles 73
Beef Mac & Cheese 64
Beef Minestrone 94
Beef Ribs 74
Beef with Peas and Corn 69
Beef with Spinach 68
Beefy Chili 93
Beefy Vegetable Soup 88
Beer Sausages 66
BLT Chicken Salad 22
Braised Oxtails 74
Braised Pork Belly 24
Breakfast Cauliflower Hash 17
Breakfast Meatloaf 16
Breakfast Pizza 11
Breakfast Pork and Avocado Mix 13
Breakfast Sweet Pepper Hash 11
Breakfast Sweet Pepper Rounds 16
Breakfast Veggie Casserole 12
Breakfast Veggie Salad 13
Brisket & Onions 75
Broccoli Cheese Casserole 86
Brunch Florentine 86
Brussels Sprouts Curry 78
Butter Pork Ribs 42

C

Cabbage Steaks 33
Carne Asada 23
Cauliflower Bites 39
Cauliflower Bolognese 83

Cauliflower Casserole 34
Cauliflower Rice 35
Cheddar Jalapeno Breakfast Sausages 13
Cheese and Mushroom Stuffed Chicken Rolls 28
Cheese Sticks 39
Cheese Stuffed and Pesto Eggplants 27
Cheeseburger & Bacon Pie 71
Cheesy Cauliflower Chowder w/ Bacon 95
Chicken & Corn Chowder 54
Chicken & Pumpkin Chili 52
Chicken Basque 51
Chicken Bites 38
Chicken Butter Mushrooms 86
Chicken Cordon Bleu Soup 53
Chicken Curry 51
Chicken Dipped in Tomatillo Sauce 61
Chicken Enchilada Casserole 50
Chicken Ginger Curry 62
Chicken Noodle Soup 50
Chicken Parmesan Soup 53
Chicken Roux Gumbo 59
Chicken Thighs with Vegetables 60
Chicken with Lemon Parsley Butter 61
Chicken with Mint Garlic Sauce & Lentils 56
Chili Verde 25
Chili Walnuts 40
Chinese Broccoli 32
Chocolate Cake 102
Chocolate Cheese Cake 100
Chocolate Peanut Butter Cups 99
Chunky Chicken Salsa 59
Cider-Braised Chicken 59
Clam Chowder 48
Classic Pork Adobo 67
Coconut Cilantro Curry Shrimp 46
Coconut Raspberry Cake 103
Coconut Yogurt 100
Cream of Broccoli-Cauliflower Soup 94
Cream of Zucchini Soup 96
Creamy Chicken Soup 91
Creamy Salmon and Dill 30
Creamy Vegan Broccoli Soup 28
Crème Brulee 100
Crustless Spinach Quiche 89
Curried Cauliflower 27
Curry Cauliflower 35

D

Delicious Garden Frittata 85
Delicious Pumpkin Custard 101
Delightful Dal 81
Dijon Chicken 60

E
- Egg and Broccoli Casserole 85
- Eggplant Bread 39
- Eggplant Gratin 36
- Eggplant Pate with Breadcrumbs 14

F
- Figs and Goat Cheese-Stuffed Chicken 22
- Fire Roasted Tomato Soup 87
- Fish Curry 44
- Flourless Chocolate Brownies 99

G
- Garlic Butter Turkey Breasts 29
- Garlic Cauliflower Steaks 35
- Garlic Shrimp 47
- Ginger Steak Broccoli 21

H
- Ham + Pumpkin Soup 95
- Ham Pitta Pockets 16
- Hamburger Style Stuffing 67
- Healthy Low Carb Walnut Zucchini Bread 17
- Honey Garlic Chicken 54
- Hoppin' John 80
- Hungarian Mushroom Soup 27

I
- Indian Style Cardamom Pork 68
- Italian Meatballs & Zoodles 72
- Italian Meatloaf 72
- Italian Ragu 75

J
- Jackfruit Carnitas 77
- Jambalaya 78

L
- Lamb and Cabbage 66
- Lamb with Mint & Green Beans 69
- Lavender and Orange Lamb 66
- Lemon Blueberry Cake 101
- Lemon Dill Halibut 46
- Lemon Pepper Tilapia 48
- Lime Chicken with Savoy Cabbage 21
- Low Carb Seafood and Sausage Gumbo 31
- Low-Carb Hash Brown Breakfast Casserole 18

M
- Mahi Mahi Taco Wraps 43
- Maple Chicken & Veggies 52
- Mashed Cauliflower 33
- Meaty Cauliflower Lasagna 25
- Mediterranean Fresh Tuna 30
- Mexican Chicken Soup 91
- Mexican Lamb Fillet 64
- Middle Eastern Lamb Zucchini Casserole 21
- Mississippi Pot Roast 75
- Mixed Nuts 38
- Moroccan Chicken 55
- Moroccan Chickpea Stew 81
- Moroccan Eggplant Mash 36
- Mushroom Stew 33
- Mushroom-Kale Stroganoff 79

N
- Nutritious Burrito Bowl 15

O
- Onion Broccoli Quiche 19
- Orange Chicken 57

P
- Paprika Almonds 38
- Paprika Chicken 61
- Paprika Shrimp 10
- Peanut Butter Pudding 100
- Pecans Bowl 41
- Peppercorn Short Ribs 24
- Poached Salmon 48
- Pork Bites 40
- Pork Breakfast Sausages 11
- Pork Ragu With Basil 68
- Potato Breakfast Mix 12
- Pumpkin and Coconut Soup 89

Q
- Quinoa Chicken Primavera 56
- Quinoa Curry 15

R
- Raspberry Yogurt 98
- Ratatouille 82
- Red Beans with the Sweet Peas 14
- Rice Pudding with Mixed Berries 98
- Rotisserie Chicken 62

S
- Salmon with Creamy Lemon Sauce 44
- Salmon with Lemon-Caper Sauce 45
- Saucy Duck 58
- Sausage Dip 42
- Sautéed Bell Peppers 37
- Shredded Pork Chili 93
- Shrimp in Marinara Sauce 47
- Shrimp Scampi 43
- Shrimp Tacos 44
- Shrimps Alfredo 30
- Simple Pork Chop Casserole 65
- Sloppy Joe Filling 79
- Slow Cooker Spaghetti Squash 32
- Soy-Ginger Steamed Pompano 49
- Spicy Barbecue Shrimp 45
- Spicy Italian Sausage and Zucchini Noodles 24
- Spicy Pepper Chicken Soup 92
- Succulent Lamb 70
- Sweet Spicy Chicken 53
- Sweet-and-Sour Tempeh 80

T
- Tandoori Salmon with Fresh Cucumber Salad 26

Tarragon Lamb & Beans 70
Tasty Greek Style Breakfast 20
Tasty Lemon Cake 102
Tasty Short Ribs 29
Tex-Mex Taco Filling 82
Thai Chicken Curry 63
Thai-Inspired Chicken Soup 91
The Ultimate Bacon Meatloaf 28
Thyme Sausage Squash 20
Tomato Salmon Meatballs 41
Tomato Soup 96
Tomatoes Aubergines 84
Turkey + Herbs Soup 92
Turkey Meatballs 41

V

Vanilla Pancakes 10
Vegan Cauliflower Rice and Beans 83
Vegetable Cheese Frittata 87
Vegetable Korma (Stew) 96
Vegetarian Tikka Masala 89
Veggie Turkey Smash 10

Z

Zucchini Gratin 36
Zucchini Lasagna 88
Zucchini Pasta 32